IMMUNITY BOOSTING FUNCTIONAL FOODS TO COMBAT COVID-19

Throughout the world people are restless to find out the ways that can minimize the risk of present outbreak of COVID-19 pandemic. It is considered that healthy eating habit is one of the remedial ways against this. The people who are weak in immunity are prone to severe attack of COVID-19. Functional foods are those foods which have health beneficial role beyond its basic nutrition. So, functional foods which can improve the immunity of the people,are helpful to combat COVID-19. The book 'Immunity Boosting Functional Foods to Combat COVID-19' contains seventeen chapters which describe immunity boosting effect of some functional foods/food ingredients such as different medicinal plants, herbs, fruits, vegetables, seeds, dairy products, probiotics, vitamins, minerals, etc. The book may be helpful to common people and health professionals as well as scientists, teachers, scholars and students.

Dr. Apurba Giri is currently working as Assistant Professor & Head, Dept. of Nutrition, and Coordinator, Dept. of Food Processing, Mugberia Gangadhar Mahavidyalaya. He did B.Tech (WBUAFS), M.Tech (KVAFSU) and Ph.D (NDRI) in Dairy Tech. and Post-Doc (IIT Kharagpur) in Food Tech. He worked as Technical Officer at City Dairy, Howrah and Sr. Officer at Banas Dairy, Gujarat. He has presented his Post-Doctoral work at Denmark Technical University with the help of UGC International Travel Grant. He is life member of World Science Congress, Indian Dairy Association, Dairy Technology Society of India, Association of Food Scientists and Technologists (India), The Indian Science Congress Association and Nutrition Society of India.

IMMUNITY BOOSTING FUNCTIONAL FOODS TO COMBAT COVID-19

Editor

Apurba Giri

B.Tech(WBUAFS), M.Tech(KVAFSU),
Ph.D(NDRI), Post-Doc(IIT-Kharagpur);
Assistant Professor and Head, Dept. of Nutrition;
Coordinator, Dept. of Food Processing;
Mugberia Gangadhar Mahavidyalaya,
[College with Potential for Excellence (UGC);
Star College (DBT, GoI); Affiliated to Vidyasagar University]
Bhupatinagar, Purba Medinipur-721425, West Bengal, India

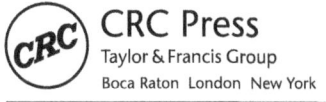

CRC Press
Taylor & Francis Group
Boca Raton London New York

CRC Press is an imprint of the
Taylor & Francis Group, an **informa** business

NARENDRA PUBLISHING HOUSE
DELHI (INDIA)

First published 2022
by CRC Press
2 Park Square, Milton Park, Abingdon, Oxon, OX14 4RN

and by CRC Press
6000 Broken Sound Parkway NW, Suite 300, Boca Raton, FL 33487-2742

CRC Press is an imprint of Informa UK Limited

British Library Cataloguing-in-Publication Data
A catalogue record for this book is available from the British Library

Library of Congress Cataloging-in-Publication Data
A catalog record has been requested

ISBN: 978-1-032-15123-6 (hbk)
ISBN: 978-1-003-24260-4 (ebk)

DOI: 10.1201/9781003242604

Dedicated To

All My Respected Teachers

CONTENTS

PREFACE

We are very much experienced that the disease COVID-19 which is originated from Wohan city of China in December, 2019, has spread all over the world and has made it pandemic. The COVID-19 pandemic has taken several lives, hampered academic system, disturbed the people's way of income generation and declined the world economy. Besides it made huge pressure to the health systems.

It has been reported that to protect against the spread of this disease some precautions may be taken - such as using mask, hand sanitizer, washing hand with soap frequently, not to go outside of home except any essential work etc. However, there is no particular treatment or medicine against this disease. It may be assumed that vaccination may be ultimate solution against this highly contagious disease. But, we have to keep in mind that the virus mutates, and may overcome the vaccine effect. Due to the RNA virus, the antigenic structure is altered frequently and that make difficult to develop a successful vaccine.

On the other hand, it has been considered that physical exercise and healthy eating habit are two effective remedial ways to fight against this disease as both enhances the body immunity. The people who are weak in immunity are prone to attack COVID-19. Functional foods are those foods which have health beneficial role beyond its basic nutrition. In this direction, functional foods which can improve the immunity of the people, are helpful to combat COVID-19. In this book 'Immunity Boosting Functional Foods to Combat COVID-19', several functional foods or food ingredients, their mechanism of immune enhancing properties and use in food products have been discussed through seventeen chapters written by eminent authors.

There are several medicinal plants which have significant role for immunity boosting such as Ashwagandha, Tulsi, Shatavari, Giloy, Aloe vera, Amla, Neem, licorice, garlic, ginger, turmeric, rosemary, black cumin, cinnamon, sage, thyme, fenugreek, peppermint, black pepper, clove etc. Angiotensin-converting enzyme 2 (ACE2) protein acts as receptor for virus's spike protein and gives provision for infection of our body. The ingredients which contain ACE inhibitory peptides, protect to produce ACE2 in our body. COVID-19 has been shown to engage the host cell ACE2 through its spike protein. It was noticed that specific compound of different medicinal plants detaches the binding interface of ACE2.

Fruits like berries and Dragon fruit and vegetables such as mushroom, broccoli also enhance body immunity due to its immunity enhancing bioactive components. It has been reported that green tea has role in immune-modulation that is mediated both through innate and adaptive immune responses. Probiotic bacteria have also been identified to have immunomodulatory role. It play a positive role in host defense mechanisms, which may include regulation of invasive bacterial translocation and the production of specific and non-specific immune responses.

Fermented milk products (as contain lactic acid bacteria and probiotic bacteria) and cheese (due to lactic acid bacteria and renneting) contain ACE inhibitory bioactive peptides. Due to this bioactive peptide, consuming cheese and fermented milk products may protect us from severe attack of corona virus.

It has been noticed that whey protein of the milk and milk product also contains very active ACE inhibitory peptide. Besides, it comprises of different fractions such as β-lactoglobulin, α-lactalbumin, immunoglobulin etc. and they have effective role to immune modulating effects for human body with different mechanisms. In addition to, food components like some vitamins (D, E, C, B6, B9, B12), some minerals (Zn, Se, Mg) have immune enhancing role.

We have to keep in mind that prevention is better than cure, even less expensive. In this direction functional foods may protect our life from the severity of this disease after attack. People have to aware about these functional foods. More researches have to be conducted on the effect of these functional foods against this disease. I hope the book will be helpful to common people and health professionals as well as scientists, teachers, scholars and students.

Apurba Giri
Editor

ACKNOWLEDGEMENTS

This book 'Immunity Boosting Functional Foods to Combat COVID-19' is a collection of papers presented in the International Webinar "Strategies to Boost Immunity by Functional Foods to Combat Covid-19" held on 15th July, 2020. The webinar was organized by the Department of Food Processing in collaboration with Dept. of Nutrition & Research Cell, Mugberia Gangadhar Mahavidyalaya, Bhupatinagar, Purba Medinipur, West Bengal. This book also includes some invited papers related to the topic of the webinar.

Immunity power is an important mechanism of human body to combat external harmful virus, bacteria, fungi, etc. To build our immune system effectively, we need to take food with proper recommended nutritional elements. We know the six basic nutritional elements are carbohydrate, protein, fat, vitamin, minerals and water. All these elements should be in our diet with good proportion. These elements with appropriate proportion in our diet could prevent malnutrition by building proper immune system in human body. Hence, we should take lot of, fresh fruits and vegetables, nuts, seeds, probiotic etc. apart from normal food like rice, bread, pulses, meat. Boosting immune system is now specially, very important issue during this COVID world. At present about 110 million people are affected by novel Corona virus around the globe and death toll reaches to above 2.4 million (20.02.2021). However I think we should maintain ICMR Protocol like using mask, creating social distaining, washing our hands and mouth and Yoga activities for combating this pandemic.

This book will extend the mental horizon of the readers by thoughtful information, because knowledge is a perpetuating and propagating process which needs continuous updating by way of mutual discussions. Hope this book will greatly enrich the interested readers and policy makers of the programme. Also it will be helpful to the researchers around the world.

It is my great pleasure that the Food Processing Department of our college has organized this type of webinar in Collaboration with our Research Cell and Nutrition Department. This book is a joint endeavor of eminent academicians and distinguished scholars to whom we owe our respect and gratitude.

We are grateful to respected Dr. Maria Leonor Silva, Assistant Professor, Centro de Investigação Interdisciplinar Egas Moniz, Cooperativa de Ensino Superior Egas Moniz, Portugal, Dr. Alexandra Bernardo, Associate Professor, Centro de

Investigação Interdisciplinar Egas Moniz, Cooperativa de Ensino Superior Egas Moniz, Portugal, Dr. Narayana, Senior Lecturer, Department of Animal Science, University of Ruhuna, Srilanka, Prof. Antony Gomes, Ex-Professor & UGC-Emeritus, UGC-BSR Fellow, Dept. of Physiology, Calcutta University, Kolkata, India, Dr. Subrota Hati, Assistant Professor, Dept. Dairy Microbiology, SMC College of Dairy Sci., Anand Agricultural University, Anand, Gujarat, India, Ms. Koyel Pal Chowdhury Research Dietician, SSKM Hospital; Guest lecturer in Haldia Institute of Health Science, IGNOU and Bangladesh Academy of Nutrition and Dietetics for giving their valuable speech in the webinar. Beside this we are grateful to Dr. Apurba Giri, Convener of the webinar and Assistant Professor and Head, Dept. of Nutrition and Department of Food Processing of the college and the Editor of this book, Dr. Bidhan Chandra Samanta, Joint Convener of the webinar and Coordinator of Research Cell and Associate Professor and Head, Department of Chemistry of the college, my colleagues, researchers who have encouraged and advised us from time to time in connection with this work. We would like to express our heartfelt thanks to all the participants, resource persons, and paper presenters of the webinar and also thanks to all the eminent thinkers who have contributed their papers for this publication. Our thanks are also to honourable members of Governing Body, Mugberia Gangadhar Mahavidyalaya, our non-teaching staffs, librarians, our beloved students for their kind co-operation in publishing this book.

Dr. Swapan Kumar Misra
Principal
Mugberia Gangadhar Mahavidyalaya

ACKNOWLEDGEMENTS

The book 'Immunity Boosting Functional Foods to Combat COVID-19' is the outcome of the series of lectures delivered by eminent professors, academicians, scientist and young researchers from colleges/ institutes/ universities in the One Day International Webinar on "Strategies to Boost Immunity by Functional Foods to Combat COVID-19" which was organized by Dept. of Food Processing in collaboration with Dept. of Nutrition & Research Cell, Mugberia Gangadhar Mahavidyalaya on 15st July, 2020. Beside this some of the invited articles related to the theme of webinar are included in this book.

I am highly indebted to Dr. Swapan Kumar Misra, Principal, Mugberia Gangadhar Mahavidyalaya for his encouragement and support to publish this book.

I thank to my guide Dr. SK Kanawjia, Retired-Principal Scientist, Dept. of Dairy Technology, National Dairy Research Institue, Karnal, Haryana for his valuable advice.

I thank to Dr. Maria Leonor Silva, Dr. Alexandra Bernardo, Dr. Narayana, Prof. Antony Gomes, Dr. Subrota Hati, and Ms. Koyel Pal Chowdhury for their valuable speech in the webinar.

I am extremely grateful to - Dr. Bidhan Chandra Samanta, Coordinator, Research Cell, Assistant Professor and Head, Dept. of Chemistry and Dr. Kalipada Maity, IQAC Coordinator, Assistant Professor and Head, Dept. of Mathematics of Mugberia G. Mahavidyalaya and Prof. Anil Kumar Chauhan, Professor, Dept. of Dairy Science and Food Technology, Institute of Agricultural Sciences, Banaras Hindu University, for their valuable advice.

I also wish to extend my thanks to all teachers of Dept. of Food Processing and Dept. of Nutrition - Ms. Sucheta Sahoo, Ms. Monalisa Roy, Mr. Sayan Das, Ms. Sruti Mandal, Ms. Moumita Samanta, Ms. Pranati Bera, Ms. Keya Dash, Ms. Rikta Jana, Mr. Prabir Jana, Mr. Tanmoy Giri and Lab attendant Mr. Prabal Das and all students of Dept. of Food Processing and Dept. of Nutrition for their help.

I also wish to extend my thanks to all the authors of this book for constant support to publish the book soon.

I am extremely grateful to all of my respected teachers throughout my academic life for sharing their knowledge and support.

Without the unfailing love and support of my family members – my parents, my uncle and aunt, my brothers and sisters, this work would not have been possible. In addition, the care, love, patience, and understanding of my wife and lovely son and daughter have been of inestimable encouragement and help.

I also express my gratitude to all the eminent contributors. I apologize if I inadvertently missed acknowledging my gratitude to anyone else.

Editor
Dr. Apurba Giri
Assistant Professor and Head, Department of Nutrition;
Coordinator, Dept. of Food Processing;
Mugberia Gangadhar Mahavidyalaya,
Bhupatinagar, West Bengal, India
E-mail: apurbandri@gmail.com

Immunity Boosting Functional Foods to Combat COVID-19, Pages: 1–25
Edited by: Apurba Giri
Copyright © 2021, Narendra Publishing House, Delhi, India

C H A P T E R - 1

POTENTIAL APPLICATIONS OF IMMUNE BOOSTING MEDICINAL PLANTS IN FUNCTIONAL FOODS TO COMBAT COVID-19

Narayana NMNK

*Senior Lecturer, Faculty of Agriculture, University of Ruhuna,
Mapalana, Kmburupitiya-81100, Sri Lanka
E-mail: nayana@ansci.ruh.ac.lk*

ABSTRACT

The novel corona virus disease COVID-19 which is caused by Severe Acute Respiratory Syndrome Coronavirus-2 (SARS-CoV-2) became a pandemic causing a huge loss to the lives of the people and to the global economic situation while imposing a significant pressure on the health structures of the nations worldwide. Immunocompromized people are more vulnerable to the infection and are at high risk of death. In the absence of an effective antiviral drug or a vaccine, alternative prophylactic and therapeutic solutions are essentially needed to be used to save the lives of the people from this disaster. The article highlighted the possibilities of utilizing medicinal plants rich in phytochemicals which are having proven immunomodulatory and antiviral activity in developing novel functional foods with acceptable consumer appeal to be used in reducing the risk of SARS CoV-2 infection by strengthening the immune system of the individual and complement the therapeutic measures taken against the disease. Innovative functional foods made by fortification of medicinal plants have a great promise to improve the general health and immensely help the general public against the viral infections such as COVID-19. Nevertheless, more evidences are required through controlled clinical trials to support the safety and efficacy of the functional foods fortified with medicinal plants.

Keywords: Antiviral, Coronavirus, Functional foods, Immune boosting, Medicinal plants, Phytochemicals

INTRODUCTION

Highly contagious novel corona virus disease, COVID-19 which was reported to be originated in the Wuhan city, Hubei Province of China during late 2019, has spread in an unprecedented manner all over the world within a short period of time causing a huge loss, not only to the lives of the people but also to the world economy creating a global crisis. It imposes a significant pressure on the health systems of the countries worldwide. COVID-19 is caused by a RNA virus and was named as Severe Acute Respiratory Syndrome Coronavirus-2 (SARS-CoV-2) (Gorbalenya et al., 2020). As of 15th September 2020, a total of 2,95,28,057 confirmed COVID-19 cases were reported while 9,34,230 were succumbed to death affecting 213 countries around the world (www.worldometer.info, 2020). However, actual number of infected people might be higher than the reported since, many in the population shows no symptoms. Radiating spread of this disease throughout the world is due mainly to the increased global travel of the people.

In the absence of a known cure or a treatment, the best way is to find alternative solutions to control this pandemic while gradually getting into the normal life until an effective anti-viral therapy and/or preventive vaccine has successfully been developed. Nevertheless, it is essential to keep in mind that the viruses mutate, hampering and overcoming the drug effect, which is also the case of SARS-CoV-2, the novel coronavirus. It is reported that, SARS-CoV has very high mutation rate (Ahmad et al., 2020). Especially for the RNA viruses, the antigenic structure is altered frequently and hence, developing a successful vaccine is a difficult task. Even though a vaccine is successfully developed, it could be less or ineffective when there is a change to the antigenic structure in the existing virus (Mousa, 2017).

Therefore, taking measures to control and prevent the risk of infection is important in managing the current problem of COVID-19. Among the several possible alternatives, taking healthy foods rich in functional ingredients to strengthen the immune system is one of the promising practices that could be recommended because a healthy immune system is vital to protect our body from the invading pathogens including viruses. Some plants especially the medicinal plants contain immunomodulatory phytochemicals which can be incorporated to develop functional foods. Some of the phytochemicals have exhibited broad spectrum antiviral activity for the viruses that shows resistance for the drugs. Those are due to the multifunctional components possess by these plants (Tolo et al., 2006). In this context the foods fortified with medicinal plants/their extracts/powders/essential oils which are having promising immunomodulatory and antiviral effects are of significant importance to fight against COVID-19. Chojnacka *et al.* (2020) reported that use of plant derived compounds and plant preparations in functional food development is relatively fast because the raw materials i.e. herbs and plants are of natural origin and are already approved for human consumption worldwide.

With the above introduction, the objective of this paper is to compile the information on different medicinal plants with promising immunomodulatory and antiviral properties in general and on COVID-19 in particular, that are having potential applications in functional food developments with favourable consumer appeal.

SARS-CoV-2 and COVID-19

SARS-CoV-2 the virus responsible for the COVID-19 disease is a RNA virus of the family *coronaviridae* (sub family *Coronavirinae*) and its lineage is similar to the coronaviruses that causes SARS but genetically distinct (Dhama *et al.*, 2020). It has a spike like projections on its enveloped surface giving it a crown like appearance and hence the name coronavirus (Kumar *et al.*, 2020; Singhal, 2020). Zhou *et al.* (2020) reported that the virus binds via viral structural spike (S) protein with angiotensin-converting enzyme 2 (ACE 2) receptor and invade the host cell primarily through endocytosis. SARS-CoV-2 virus transmitted from person to person by multiple means such as aerosols, droplets and fomites (Wang and Du, 2020) by contacting with the eyes, nose and the mouth. Symptoms of COVID-19 include fever, cough, myalgia or fatigue and less frequently headache, hemoptysis and diarrhea (Huang *et al.*, 2020). In a study carried out in UK, Menni *et al.* (2020) reported that loss of taste and smell is also a strong predictor of having been infected with COVID-19. However, the clinical features have a wide range from being no signs or asymptomatic to severe respiratory disorders that need intensive care under hospitalization. Tian (2020) reported that SARS-CoV-2 has shown less severe pathogenesis compared to the SARS-CoV and MERS-CoV, but high transmission competence as evidence by the continuous increase in the confirmed cases worldwide. Further, SARS-CoV-2 has unique characteristics. One such character is around 80% of the affected people shows no symptoms (Day, 2020) and they act as silent carriers and spread the disease. Also there is no guarantee that the patients recovered from the disease are protected from the next time infection (WHO, 2020). Those are the reasons for the high transmission competence of this virus. To date no effective vaccine or antiviral drug is available to treat COVID-19.

Healthy Immune System to Fight Against Diseases

Immune system is a complicated defense system and act to protect the host against invading harmful microorganisms such as bacteria, viruses, fungi, parasites etc. and malignant cells (Calder and Kew, 2002; Venkatalakshmi et al., 2016). Therefore, a healthy immune system is an important weapon to fight against pathogens including viruses such as SARS-CoV-2 that causes the COVID-19. However, it is well documented that the immune-competence of a person is affected by many factors such as age (Castelo-Branco and Soveral, 2014; Scepanovic et al., 2018), sex (Oertelt-Prigione, 2012), genetic variability (Scepanovic et al., 2018), stress (Pruett, 2003), alcohol/drug abuse (Friedman et al., 2003), malnutrition (França et al., 2009), environmental pollution (Venkatalakshmi et al., 2016), lifestyle (Venkatalakshmi et al., 2016) etc. With respect to the COVID-19 pandemic, Wu et al. (2020) reported that the older age patients had both Acute Respiratory Distress Syndrome (ARDS) and death than the others and one of the main reasons is less rigorous immune system that they possess. Therefore, enhancing immunity is definitely one of the ways medical practitioners all over the world have been using to treat this deadly disease (Balkrishna, 2020). Getting a healthy diet is one of the ways among many others such as having adequate quality sleep, stress management, doing regular physical activity and relaxation practices etc. which help to keep the immune system strong. Panyod et al. (2020) mentioned that since treating influenza with large amounts of vitamin C, which is known to boost immunity, has been practiced for decades; it might be an effective nutritional treatment for COVID-19 as well. It has already been reported that, high doses of vitamin C have been administered to the COVID-19 patients in China and some other places in the world and has shown promising results (Balkrishna, 2020).

Medicinal Plants as a Mine of Phytochemicals

Plants are considered as biosynthetic laboratory of phytochemicals (Venkatalakshmi et al., 2016) such as alkaloids, flavonoids, glycosides, steroids, polyphenols, polysaccharides, vitamins, tannins, coumarins, gums, terpenes, terpenoides etc. (Okwu, 2004; Mittal et al., 2014; Venkatalakshmi et al., 2016). Phytochemicals are secondary metabolites that do not essentially needed for the survival of the plant but produced as a response to external stimuli such as infection, changes in the nutrition, climate etc. and accumulated only in certain parts of the plant (Verpoorte et al., 1999). They serve as the natural defense system for the host plant (Venkatalakshmi et al., 2016). Medicinal plants which are rich in phytochemicals have been used from prehistoric times as natural medicines for prophylactic and therapeutic purposes as a safer alternative (Lin *et al.*, 2014; Mittal *et al.*, 2014; Ahmad *et al.*, 2020). Medicinal plants contain properties or compounds which can be used for therapeutic purposes or those that synthesize metabolites to produce useful drugs. Immune-modulatory and antimicrobial (including antiviral, antibacterial, antifungal, antiprotozoal, anthelmintic) activity are few of the potentials among many others such as anti-oxidant, anti-diabetic, memory enhancing, cholesterol lowering, anticancer, anti diarrheal, anti inflammatory, anti hypertensive, anti allergic, anti asthmatic, anti arthritic, adaptogenic, anti stress etc. possess by phytochemicals present in these plants (Goel *et al.*, 2010; Pavaraj *et al.,* 2011; Hemalatha *et al.*, 2011; Venkatalakshmi *et al.*, 2016; Vinaya *et al.*, 2017).

Utilization of Medicinal Plants for the Fortification of Functional Foods

Haslberger *et al.* (2020) in their mini review, referring to WHO expert report on clinical studies on combination treatments for SARS which has immerged earlier, mentioned that functional foods possess a huge possibility for avoiding the mechanisms of viral infection and altering immune responses. The functional food concept was initially introduced by Japanese scientists in 1984, and in Japan, those foods have been marketed as "Foods for Specified Health Use" (FOSHU). Roberfroid (2000) defined functional foods as the foods which are used to enhance certain physiological functions of the body in order to prevent or even to cure diseases. According to Hasler and Brown (2009), functional foods are defined as whole, fortified, enriched or enhanced foods that provide health benefits beyond the provision of essential nutrients, when consumed at efficacious levels as part of a varied diet on a regular basis. López-Varela *et al.* (2011) mentioned that even though natural foods have been considered as functional foods, only the foods which have undergone a methodology is preferred as functional foods. Therefore, the definition of functional food is a debatable issue. However, all the functional foods ultimately provide health benefits further to the basic nutrition that they provide. Even though functional foods are healthy, taste and pleasure are also important for them to be successful in the market, since the majority of the consumers' leading food choice motive was identified as the taste (Narayana *et al.*, 2020; Zezelj *et al.*, 2012). Further, it is highlighted that functional foods are foods and not drugs and required to be consumed in normal amounts with the normal diet.

Functional foods developed by incorporating phytochemicals rich medicinal plants, plant parts and extracts play a significant role in the market and are having a huge demand and a potential in this era of COVID-19 than ever before. Addition of herbs and spices which are having medicinal and other functional value to foods are also not new and it has been practiced from ancient times. Nevertheless, novel products, for an example, novel dairy products fortified with such medicinal plants could be developed and they give more value for the money spends by health conscious consumers while helping to protect their lives. A variety of medicinal plants with immunomodulatory and potential antiviral activity have been identified by the scientific community (Agarwal *et al.*, 1999; Cinatl *et al.*, 2003; Goel *et al.*, 2010; Balasubramani *et al.*, 2011; Hemalatha *et al.*, 2011; Mondal *et al.*, 2011; Pavaraj *et al.*, 2011; Jayati *et al.*, 2013; Balkrishna, 2020;) which are having potential applications in the functional food industry. They could be recommended to reduce the risk of SARS CoV-2 infection by strengthening the immune system of an individual and complement the therapeutic measures taken against the disease.

Medicinal Plants of Significance for Functional Food Development to Combat COVID-19

Ashwagandha (*Withania somnifera* L.)

Ashwagandha (*Withania somnifera*) has been utilized in traditional medicine for more than 3000 years and the bioactive compounds derived from this valuable plant are used in prevention and treatment of various diseases (Gill *et al.*, 2019; Balkrishna, 2020). It has been stated that *W. somnifera* possess many beneficial health properties such as antioxidant (Chaurasia *et al.*, 2000), antimicrobial including antiviral (Pant *et al.*, 2012), immunomodulatory (El-Boshy *et al.*, 2013), anti-inflammatory (Chandra *et al.*, 2012), anticancer (Wadhwa *et al.*, 2013), adaptogenic, cardio protective (Dhuley, 2000) etc. Reported health benefits are due to the existence of many phytochemical compounds such as steroidal lactones (withanolides, withaferins), steroidal alkaloids, saponins, flavonoids, phenols, carbohydrates, glycosides, phytosterols, terpenoides etc. present in this valuable medicinal herb (Tiwari *et al.*, 2014; Swaminathan and Santhi, 2019). Tiwari *et al.* (2014) reported that steroidal lactones and steroidal alkaloids present in this herb are mainly responsible for the health benefits that it possess.

Pant *et al.* (2012) studied the antiviral activity of *W. somnifera* root extract against Infectious Bursal Disease (IBD) virus replication. They have used cytopathic effect reduction assay for the study and showed that *W. somnifera* has a promising effect against IBD virus. El-Boshy *et al.* (2013) carried out a study to find the effect of *W. somnifera* extract on immunological, hematological and biochemical parameters in guinea pigs against *E. coli* attack. They have shown that *W. somnifera* has the ability to correct immunological, hematological and biochemical alterations caused as response of infection. Molecular docking simulations predicted the therapeutic significance of withanone, one of the active withanolides of *W. somnifera*, which is capable of binding to the substrate binding pockets of SARS-CoV-2-M^{pro}, a highly conserved protein of SARS-CoV-2 (Kumar *et al.*, 2020). Further, Balkrishna (2020) also showed that withanone docked well in the binding interface of ACE2-RBD (of SARS-CoV-2) complex and on simulation move slightly towards the center of the interface. Author proposed that such an interaction would block or weaken the COVID-19 entry as well as the infectivity.

The possibilities of using *W. somnifera* in functional food applications have been reported. Anita *et al.* (2017) successfully optimized a cookie formulation with *W. somnifera* leaf powder using response surface methodology. Indu and Awasthi (2008) developed cereal-legume based biscuit fortified with *W. somnifera* root powder and concluded that up to 5% powder can be fortified without affecting organoleptic quality of the biscuit which have high mineral content. Gill *et al.* (2019) reported that a dose of 3-6 mg of leaves and/or roots of *W. somnifera* is recommended to be incorporated in functional food formulations in powder form or as it is. Dairy products also have been developed by incorporating *W. somnifera* (Viswaroopan *et al.*, 2015; Singh *et al.*, 2018). Still, great opportunities are available to develop innovative functional food products to get the advantage of this valuable herb in disease prevention in this era of COVID-19.

Tulsi/holy basil (*Ocimum sanctum* L.)

Tulsi (*Ocimum sanctum* L.) which is known in Ayurveda as "the queen of herbs" (Singh *et al.*, 2010) has a wide array of health benefits (Cohen, 2014). Antimicrobial (including antiviral) (Jayati *et al.*, 2013), antioxidant (Yadav and Shukla, 2014), anti-asthmatic (Vinaya *et al.*, 2017), anti-carcinogenic (Karthikeyan *et al.*, 1999), immunomodulatory (Goel *et al.*, 2010; Pavaraj *et al.*, 2011; Hemalatha *et al.*, 2011; Mondal *et al.*, 2011) are few of the scientifically proven health benefits among many others of*O. sanctum*. These benefits are attributable to the high amount of phenolic compounds and antioxidant properties present in the plant (Wangcharoen and Morasuk, 2007). Borah and Biswas (2018) reported that *O. sanctum* contains various phytochemicals including carbohydrate, tannin, flavonoids, saponins, glycosides, terpenoids, fatty acids and phenols in their leaf extract. In Ayurveda, *O. sanctum* is widely used to treat many health ailments such as infections, skin diseases, cold, cough, malaria fever, hepatic disorders etc. (Hemalatha *et al.*, 2011). Daily consumption of this herb is known to prevent diseases and to improve the general health. Further, broad spectrum of antimicrobial activity of *O. sanctum* is important for many applications including food preservation (Cohen, 2014).

Pavaraj *et al.* (2011) used different concentrations of *O. sanctum* extract on common carp (*Cyprinus carpio* L.) fingerlings to study the immunity development against heat damaged bacterial pathogen *Aeromonas hydrophila* as an antigen and found that both specific as well as non-specific immunity was enhanced at 10 ppm level of the extract. Further, the authors mentioned that low concentration of plant extract is sufficient to exhibit an immunostimulant effect and hence its use is cost effective. Goel *et al.* (2010) carried out a study to find out the effect of aqueous extract of *O. sanctum* leaves on interleukin-2 (IL-2) cytokine production *in vitro* and *in vivo* and on routine blood parameters and T& B lymphocytes in peripheral blood. They have shown that aqueous *O. sanctum* leaves extract have a stimulatory effect on T & B lymphocytes particularly on Th1 subset of lymphocytes as indicated by enhancement in IL-2 production confirming its use as a potent immunomodulator. Hemalatha *et al.* (2011) in their study to find out the immunomodulatory activity and Th1/Th2 cytokine response of *O. sanctum* using albino mice concluded that *O. sanctum* is a potential immunomodulator since it possess the ability to alter the NF-κB activity. Significant immunomodulatory role was reported by Mondal *et al.* (2011) who studied the effect of ethanolic extract of *O. sanctum* on healthy volunteer adults using double-blind randomized cross-over trial.

Jayati *et al.* (2013) studied the *in vitro* anti-viral effect of *O. sanctum* leaf extract against the virus causing new castle disease (NCD) in poultry using chicken embryo fibroblast monolayer culture. They have reported that the leaf extract of *O. sanctum* showed a potent antiviral activity against the NCD due to the absence of cytopathic effects in monolayer and lower the haemagglutination assay (HA) titer. RNA dependent RNA polymerase (RDRP) without which viruses cannot survive was targeted using *O. sanctum* phytochemicals by Balkrishna (2020) in his *in-silico* study. Author reported that few phytochemical compounds present in *O. sanctum* hit the catalytic cleft of the RDRP and scutellarein is one of them. Accordingly, author suggested that phytochemicals in *O. sanctum* could inhibit the coronavirus replication and control its growth and spread.

O. sanctum is used traditionally in many formssuchas herbal tea, dried powder, fresh leaf, or mixed with Honey and Ghee (Amarah *et al.*, 2017). Further it has shown promising applications in other functional foods as well. Juntachote *et al.* (2006) studied the antioxidant potential of *O. sanctum* on cooked ground pork and showed that dried powder can be used as a possible natural antioxidant in food preservation. Alam *et al.* (2013) developed fibre enriched herbal biscuits using *O. sanctum* leaves and concluded that organoleptically acceptable functional biscuit can be manufactured by incorporating leaves up to a level of 1%. *O. sanctum* fortified cookies and biscuits are already available in the market as well. Even though there is a controversy of using *O. sanctum* with milk, milk based functional foods such as ice cream (Kumar *et al.*, 2013), ice lolly (Misra, 2016), yoghurt, milk drink etc. have been successfully developed using it and also commercially available. Enormous opportunity is ahead to develop different functional foods using this herb to satisfy the diversified consumer preferences especially to boost the immunity and to prevent from viral infections.

Giloy (*Tinospora cordifolia* Miers.)

T. cordifolia has been utilized in Ayurveda and traditional medicine since ancient times. The plant has variety of bioactive phytochemical compounds such as alkaloids, glycosides aliphatic compounds, diterpenoid lactones, steroids, polysaccharides, polyphenols etc. in various parts of the plant (Mittal *et al.*, 2014; Khan *et al.*, 2020). *T. cordifolia* is well recognized for its immunomodulatory effects. Among the bioactive phytochemicals, the compounds such as 11-hydroxymuskatone, N-methyle-2-pyrrolidone, N-formylannonain, cordifolioside A, magnoflorine, tinocordioside and syringing showed promising results as having immunomodulatory effects (Sharma *et al.*, 2012; Mittal *et al.*, 2014).

Immunomodulatory potential of *T. cordifolia* against IBD virus was investigated in chicken by Sachan *et al.* (2019). They showed that *T. cordifolia* significantly ($p<0.05$) increased the interferon gamma (IFN-γ), IL-2, IL-4, and IL-1 levels in the peripheral blood mononuclear cells of chicken following infection, which shows the potential of *T. cordifolia* to act as an immunomodulatory and antiviral agent due to the phytochemicals present.

Balkrishna (2020) mentioned that out of the phytochemicals reported in *T. cordifolia*, tinocordiside docked well within the ACE-RBD (of the SARS-CoV-2) complex in their *in-silico* study. Further, the author reported that in the simulated state, tinocordiside showed satisfactory binding poses within the interface of ACE2-RBD with several interacting sites. Hence the author claimed that *T. cordifolia* is a potent medicinal plant to be used for drug discovery against COVID-19 caused by SARS-CoV-2. In another *in-silico* study, Chowdhury (2020) reported that among the phytochemicals considered in *T. cordifolia*, berberine could regulate the function of viral 3CL[pro] or M[pro] protein which is a key CoV enzyme, thus have the possibility to control viral replication.

Bioactive polyphenol profiling and *in vitro* antioxidant activity of *T. cordifolia* was studied by Khan *et al.* (2020) and they mentioned that this medicinal plant has an excellent potential to be used in functional food formulations.

Licorice (*Glycyrriza glabra* L.)

Licorice (*Glycyrriza glabra*) is an extensively used medicinal plant in Ayurveda and traditional medicine from the time immemorial. It is known as 'the father of the herbal medicines' (Foster *et al.*, 2017). *G. glabra* is utilized in traditional medicine to treat a range of health complaints such as respiratory tract problems, digestive system related disorders, epilepsy, paralysis, rheumatism, cancer, malaria etc. (Batiha *et al.*, 2020) and it has vast array of biological effects such as anti-inflammatory, anti-allergic, anti-viral, antioxidant etc. (Sawant *et al.*, 2016). Wang *et al.* (2015) reported that *G. glabra* contains more than 20 triterpenoides and nearly 300 flavounoides. It contains glycyrrhizin and many other phytochemicals such as flavonoids, saponins, glycosides, tannins, steroids etc. (Sawant *et al.*, 2016).

Immunomodulatory activity of aqueous methanolic extract of *G. glabra* was studied by Hussain *et al.* (2017) against *Eimeria* species infection in broiler chickens. They have reported that the treated group showed significantly (*P<0.05*) higher dose dependent cell mediated and humoral response as compared to negative control. In the review on antiviral and antimicrobial activity of *G. glabra*, Wang *et al.* (2015) reported that among the phytochemicals identified glycyrrhizin and glycyrrhetinic acid have been reported to have potent antiviral effect. Reported phytochemicals interfere with the viral activity by many ways such as inhibition of viral gene expression and replication, reduction of adhesion force etc.

Behrad *et al.* (2009) studied the effect of *G. glabra* incorporated yoghurt on probiotic fermentation and *Helicobacter pylori* growth *in-vitro*. They have found that the addition of *G. glabra* did not change the yoghurt fermentation but inhibit the *H. pylori* showing its antimicrobial ability and possibility of utilizing in fermented functional food preparations. *G. glabra* is used in both pharmaceutical and health food sector to flavor the food and beverages and also used in tobacco industry to flavor tobacco products (Sawant *et al.*, 2016). Ishimi *et al.* (2019) reported that *G. glabra* is a highly used raw material in health foods in Japanese market.

The safety and effectiveness of *G. glabra* in health foods available in Japanese market was evaluated by Ishimi *et al.* (2019). They have detected glabridine and small amount of glycyrrhizin in those products and have mentioned that even though there is a claim that licorice has a beneficial effect on bone health in postmenopausal women, overdose of the functional foods containing licorice should be avoided by young women because of the estrogenic activity that was identified in some of the related compounds and products. Further, Deutch *et al.* (2019) reported that too much consumption of *G. glabra* will increase the blood pressure and can cause life threatening complications especially in the patients suffering from cardiovascular diseases. Therefore, even though *G. glabra* has many health benefits, overconsumption should be avoided.

Shatavari (*Asparagus racemosus* Willd.)

Shatavari (*Asparagus racemosus*) is a popular vine widely used for its medicinal value. Both leaves and roots are utilized in Ayurveda and other food preparations. Leaves are frequently used in Sri Lanka to make porridge and it is having a pleasant characteristic flavor. Therefore, *A. racemosus* has a huge potential to be used in functional food applications with acceptable consumer appeal.Shevale *et al.* (2015) reported that *A. racemosus* contains many phytochemicals such as alkaloids, glycosides, phenolic compounds, tannins, saponins, steroids, flavonoids and carbohydrates. Thakur *et al.* (2012) reported that among many phytochemicals present in *A. racemosus,* fructooligosaccharides and other polysaccharides are responsible for the immunomodulatory properties that the plant possesses. Gautam *et al.* (2009) studied the effect of standardized *A. racemosus* root aqueous extract on systemic Th1/Th2 immunity of sheep blood cells sensitized mice. They suggested that *A. racemosus* root aqueous extract has cytoprotective, immunorestorative activities with mixed Th1/Th2 response and proposed to be used as vaccine or immunoadjuvant. In a study conducted by Veena *et al.* (2014) highlighted the immunomodulatory potential of *A. racemosus* root extract fortified milk due to the increased phagocytic activity of macrophages *in vitro.*

With the view of utilizing in functional dairy product development, Veena *et al.* (2015) studied how *A. racemosus* root extract interacts with milk proteins and influences the physichochemical and functional properties of milk. They have mentioned that the addition of *A. racemosus* root extract interacted with milk proteins and had an influence on the colour, viscosity, heat stability and rennet coagulation time of fortified milk. The information generated by them is useful in developing *A. racemosus* fortified functional dairy products. Singh *et al.* (2014) optimized functional bread preparation with *A. racemosus* root powder using response surface methodology. They have reported that all the phytochemicals present in the original herb powder except flavounoides were found in the optimized bread which has a favourable consumer acceptance. Rani *et al.* (2020) developed functional biscuit fortified with *A. racemosus* root powder and they have concluded that up to 10% powder can be successfully used without compromising the taste of the biscuits with increased shelf life. In Ayurveda *A. racemosus* has been described as a safe herb for long term use and it is recommended to be used even under pregnancy and lactation (Alok *et al.*, 2013).

Garlic (*Allium sativum* L.)

Garlic (*Allium sativum* L.) has been used as a valuable medicinal plant for centuries in traditional medicine and in culinary preparations. It has a high reputation in many traditions as a prophylactic and as well as a therapeutic agent (Bayan *et al.*, 2014). *A. sativum* contains organosulfur compounds along with saponins, phenolic compounds and polysaccharides with remarkable biological and pharmacological properties (Tapiero *et al.*, 2004; Arreola *et al.*, 2015; Shang *et al.*, 2019). *A. sativum* possesses a wide array of health benefits such as anti-cancer (Li *et al.*, 2018), antibacterial (Strika *et al.*, 2016), antiviral (Mehrbod *et al.*, 2009), anti-diabetic (Eidi *et al.*, 2006), anti-hypertensive (Ashraf *et al.*, 2013), cardioprotective (Abdel-Baky and Abdel-Rahman, 2020), hepatoprotective (Ilyas *et al.*, 2011), hypolipidemic (Murthy *et al.*, 2014), antioxidant (Awan *et al.*, 2018) as well as immunomodulatory (Keiss *et al.*, 2003) Goêbiowska-Wawrzyniak *et al.*, 2004) due primarily to the presence of organosulfur compounds.

Keiss *et al.* (2003) studied the effect of *A. sativum* powder extract on cytokine expression in lipopolysaccharide activated human blood samples. They have shown that *A. sativum* can promote the anti-inflammatory environment by cytokine modulation in human blood that leads to an overall inhibition of NF-κB activity in surrounding tissues. Goêbiowska-Wawrzyniak *et al.* (2004) in a pilot investigation treated the children suffering from recurrent respiratory tract infections and mild cellular immunodeficiency with dry *A. sativum* tablets and shown that there was a significant improvement in T-lymphocyte function as well as the clinical conditions. Further, Donma and Donma (2020) reviewed the capability of the *A. sativum* to maintain the immunohomeostasis in an individual through different ways.Rouf *et al.* (2020) reported that garlic has antiviral activity not only against human and animal but also against plant viral infections. Mehrbod *et al.* (2009) investigated the antiviral activity of *A. sativum* extract against the influenza virus using Madin-Darbey Canine Kidney cell culture and showed the successful inhibitory effect of *A. sativum* extract on the virus penetration and proliferation.

While *A. sativum* is used in many culinary preparations and considered itself as a functional food and also since the phytochemical substances in it have been proposed as promising candidates for immune homeostasis and as an antiviral agent, it could be used as a effective ingredient in functional food development with high consumer appeal to be used in this era of COVID-19. In the current market, garlic fortified functional foods like bakery products such as bread, biscuits, and herbal teas, pickle, sauce etc. are already available and new ways and means in utilization of this valuable medicinal plant should be explored.

Aloe vera

Aloe vera has been utilized in traditional medicine for around 3000 years (Dagne *et al.*, 2000). Luta and McAnalley (2005) reported that on dry matter basis *A. vera* gel consists of polysaccharides (55%), sugars (17%), minerals (16%), proteins (7%), lipids (4%) and phenolic compounds (1%). According to Kahramanoglu *et al.* (2019), *A. vera* contains nearly 110 potentially active constituents which belong to 6 different classes. Among them, chromone and anthraquinone and their glycoside derivatives are of significant importance. Immunomodulatory and antiviral potential of *A. vera* was examined and proven by previous studies (Keivan *et al.*, 2007; Halder *et al.*, 2012). *A. vera* gel as well as the powder prepared from the gel is already extensively utilized in various health foods worldwide. Ahlawat and Khatkar (2011) reported that *A. vera* products are amongst the popular products in the functional foods and supplements market in USA. Even though *A. vera* gel is safe to use, aloin from the yellow exudates is reported to cause DNA damage and cancer (Lachenmeier *et al.* 2005) and therefore, *A. vera* products should be manufactured with utmost care. Apart from used in functional food applications, *A. vera* gel is used in the food applications as an edible coating to preserve fresh produce (Kahramanoglu *et al.*, 2019). Postharvest quality of the fresh produce will be protected by application of *A. vera* due to the inhibition/reduction of respiration and transpiration by these fresh produce.

Other Medicinal Plants Having Proven Immonomodulatory and Antiviral Activity with Potential Applications in Functional Foods

Apart from the medicinal plants mentioned above there is a possibility of many others with proven antiviral and immunomodulatory properties such as *Zingiber officinale* (ginger), *Curcuma longa* (turmeric), *Salvia rosmarinus* (rosemary), *Nigella sativa* (black cumin), *Cinnamomum verum* (cinnamon), *Salvia officinalis* (sage), *Thymus vulgaris* (thyme), *Houttuynia cordata, Trigonella foenum-graecum* (fenugreek), *Mentha piperita* (peppermint) etc. to be utilized in functional food applications. Some of them have already been utilized and some, experimented to be fortified in functional foods development. The health benefit of *Zingiber officinale* was documented around 2000 years ago (Caroviæ-Stanko *et al.*, 2016) and used in many food applications. Some others mentioned above are normally used in culinary preparations as spices. It has been documented that *H. cordata* which is widely used in some countries as a leafy vegetable and *N. sativa* which is widely used as a spice possess anti-SARS activity. Lau *et al.* (2008) studied the effect of aqueous extract of *H. cordata* on immunomodulatory and anti-SARS activity in mouse model. They reported that *H. cordata* act against SARS in 2 different ways, i.e. by activating cell mediated immunity to prevent viral infection and if infected, by slowing down the viral replication. They also documented that *H. cordata* water extractis not toxic to laboratory animals after the oral administration of 16 g/kg. Since *H. cordata* has a fishy smell, there is a possibility to use extracts/powders of this plant with fish and meat based functional foods. Sommer *et al.* (2020) reported that due to the existence of thymoquinone, one of the main phytochemical compounds, *N. sativa* is an effective herb which can be utilized to treat SARS-CoV-2. Thymoquinone might be potent against SARS-CoV-2 by inhibiting viral proliferation, by killing the virus, by killing bacteria associated with pneumonia and by improving the immunity (Sommer *et al.*, 2020). *N. sativa* and its essential oil have many functional food applications already (Ramadan, 2007). Since the above mentioned medicinal plants have proven antiviral and immunomodulatory activities, novel functional food products with higher consumer acceptability could be developed for the functional food market to be used by the health conscious consumers worldwide especially in this crisis situation of COVID-19 to improve their overall health and to protect from being infected.

CONCLUSION

Medicinal plants have been used since ancient times in traditional medicine as prophylactic and therapeutic agents for various health ailments. Bioactive phytochemicals derived from those plants have several different scientifically proven health benefits including immunomodulatory and antiviral properties. Optimal cultivation, harvesting, preservation and storage conditions are required to preserve the medicinal value of these medicinal plants. It is also crucial to guarantee the correct plant is used. Rigorous quality assurance measures are needed to be applied to the products not only in the functional food sector but also in any application to guarantee the product quality, safety and efficacy and thereby to ensure consumer health. Quality and quantity of bioactive phytochemicals present in the final functional food should be assured. For this, product claims are needed to be tested. The claims should be verified and certified by regulatory authorities before delivered to the market. Phytochemicals in the medicinal plants when fortified can interact with the food matrix. Therefore, thousands of years of usage cannot be taken as evidence for safety and efficacy of medicinal plants when incorporated with foods. Hence, more evidence is required through controlled clinical trials to support the safety and efficacy of the functional foods fortified with medicinal plants. Studies should also be carried out using specific food substrates under storage and food processing conditions. Functional foods with better consumer appeal developed accordingly, could be utilized as an effective means for the prevention of diseases. They could enhance the immunohomeostasis and protect the body against COVID-19. Functional foods can be recommended to enhance the immunity of the group of people who are unexposed as well as exposed to COVID-19.

REFERENCES

Abdel-Baky ES, Abdel-Rahman ON (2020) Cardioprotective effects of the garlic (*Allium sativum*) in sodium fluoride-treated rats. *The Journal of Basic and Applied Zoology* **81**:1-7. https://doi.org/10.1186/s41936-020-0140-0.

Agarwal R, Diwanay S, Patki P, Patwardhan B (1999) Studies on immunomodulatory activity of *Withania somnifera* (Ashwa gandha) extracts in experimental immune inflammation. *J Ethnopharmacol* **67**: 27–35.

Ahlawat KS, Khatkar BS (2011) Processing, food applications and safety of *Aloe vera* products: a review. *J Food Sci Technol* **48(5)**: 525–533.

Ahmad A, Rehman MU, Alkharfy KM (2020) An alternative approach to minimize the risk of coronavirus (Covid-19) and similar infections. *Eur Rev Med Pharmacol Sci* **24**: 4030-4034.

Alam MJ, Huq AKO, Prodhan UK, Talukder MU (2013) Development of Fiber Enriched Herbal Biscuits by Incorporating Tulsi Leaves on Wheat Flour: A Preliminary Study on Sensory Evaluation and Chemical Composition. *Res Rev J Herb Sci* **2(2)**: 1-5.

Alok S, Jain SK, Verma A, Kumar M, Mahor A, Sabharwal M (2013) Plant profile, phytochemistry and pharmacology of Asparagus racemosus (Shatavari): A review. *Asian Pac J Trop Dis* **3(3)**: 242-251.

Amarah U, Chatra L, Shenai P, Veena KM, Prabhu RV, Kumar V (2017) Miracle Plant- Tulsi. *World J Pharm Pharm Sci* **6(1)**: 1567-1581.

Anita S, MonishaD, Sundararajan P, Narasimman S, Bharath G (2017) Formulation of *Withania somnifera* based herbal cookies using response surface methodology. *Int Res J Pharm* **8(6)** DOI: 10.7897/2230-8407.086105.

Arreola R, Quintero-Fabián S, López-Roa RI, Flores-Gutiérrez EO, Reyes-Grajeda JP, Carrera-Quintanar L, Ortuño-Sahagún D (2015) Immunomodulation and Anti-Inflammatory Effects of Garlic Compounds. *J Immunol Res*http://dx.doi.org/10.1155/2015/401630.

Ashraf R, Khan RA, Ashraf I, Qureshi AA (2013) Effects of *Allium sativum* (Garlic) on systolic and diastolic blood pressure in patients with essential hypertension. *Pak J Pharm Sci* **26(5)**: 859-863.

Awan KA, Butt MS, Ul Haq I, Suleria HAR (2018) Investigating the Antioxidant Potential of Garlic (Allium sativum) Extracts through Different Extraction Modes. *Curr Bioact Compd* 14. DOI: 10.2174/1573407213666171024121712.

Balasubramani SP, Venkatasubramanian P, Kukkupuni SK, Patwardhan B (2011) Plant-based Rasayana drugs from Ayurveda. *Chin J Integr Med* **17**: 88–94.

Balkrishna A (2020) Indian Traditional Ayurvedic Treatment Regime for Novel Coronavirus, COVID-19. Patanjali Research Institute. Patanjali Yogpeeth Trust Haridwar, Uttarakhand, India.https://www.patanjaliresearchinstitute.com/pdf/covid-19/Patanjali_Proposal_to_Battle_COVID-19 1.pdf.

Batiha GE, Beshbishy AM, El-Mleeh A, Abdel-Daim MM, Devkota HP (2020) Traditional Uses, Bioactive Chemical Constituents, and Pharmacological and Toxicological Activities of *Glycyrrhiza glabra* L. (Fabaceae). *Biomolecules* 10 doi:10.3390/biom10030352.

Bayan L, Koulivand PH, Gorji A (2014) Garlic: a review of potential therapeutic effects. *Avicenna J Phytomed* **4(1)**: 1-14.

Behrad S, Yusof MY, Goh KL, Baba AS (2009) Manipulation of Probiotics Fermentation of Yogurt by Cinnamon and Licorice: Effects on Yogurt Formation and Inhibition of Helicobacter Pylori Growth in vitro.*World Acad Sci Eng Technol* **60**:590-594.

Borah R, Biswas SP (2018) Tulsi (Ocimum sanctum), excellent source of phytochemicals. *Int J Environ Agric Biotech* **3(5)**: 1732-1738.

Calder PC, Kew S (2002) The immune system: a target for functional foods. *Br J Nutr* **88**: S165-176.

Caroviæ-Stanko K, Petek M, Grdiša M, Pintar J, Bedekoviæ D, Æustiæ MH, Satovic Z (2016) Medicinal Plants of the Family Lamiaceae as Functional Foods – a Review *Czech J Food Sci* **34(5)**: 377–390

Castelo-Branco C, Soveral I (2014) The immune system and ageing: a review. *Gynecol Endocrinol* **30(1)**: 16-22.

Chandra S, Chatterjee P, Dey P, Bhattacharya S (2012) Evaluation of Anti-inflammatory Effect of Ashwagandha: A Preliminary Study *in vitro*. *Phcog J* **4(29)**: 47-49.

Chaurasia SS, Panda S, Kar A (2000) Withania somnifera root extract in the regulation of led induced oxidative damage in the male mouse. *Pharmacol Res* **41**: 663-666.

Chojnacka K, Witek-Krowiak A, Skrzypczak D, Mikula K, M³ynarz P (2020) Phytochemicals containing biologically active polyphenols as an effective agent against Covid-19-inducing coronavirus. *J Funct Foods* **73**. https://doi.org/ 10.1016 /j.jff.2020.104146.

Chowdhury P (2020) In silico investigation of phytoconstituents from Indian medicinal herb *Tinospora cordifolia* (giloy) against SARS-CoV-2 (COVID-19) by molecular dynamics approach. *J Biomol Struct Dyn*DOI: 10.1080/ 07391102.2020.1803968.

Cinatl J, Morgenstern B, Bauer G, Chandra P, Rabenau H, Doerr HW (2003) Glycyrrhizin, an active component of liquorice roots, and replication of SARS-associated coronavirus. *Lancet* **361**: 2045–2046

Cohen MM (2014) Tulsi-Ocimum sanctum: A herb for all reasons. *J Ayurveda Integr Med* **5 (4)**: 251-259.

Dagne E, Bisrat D, Viljoen A, Van Wyk BE (2000) Chemistry of *Aloe* Species. *Curr Org Chem* **4:** 1055–1078.

Day M (2020) Covid-19: four fifths of cases are asymptomatic, China figures indicate. BMJ 2020; 369:m1375 doi: 10.1136/bmj.m1375.

Dhama K, Sharun K, Tiwari R, Sircar S, Bhat S, Malik SY, Singh KP, Chaicumpa W, Bonilla-Aldana DK, Rodriguez-Morales AJ (2020) Coronavirus Disease 2019 – COVID-19. doi:10.20944/preprints202003.0001. **2:** 1-75.

Dhuley JN (2000) Adaptogenic and cardioprotective action of Ashwagandha in rata and frogs. *J Ethnopharmacol* **70**: 57-63.

Donma MM, Donma O (2020) The effects of *Allium sativum* on immunity within the scope of COVID-19 infection. *Med Hypotheses* 144: 109934. https:// doi.org/10.1016/j.mehy.2020. 109934.

Deutch MR, Grimm D, Wehland M, Infanger M, Krüger M (2019) Bioactive Candy: Effects of Licorice on the Cardiovascular System. *Foods* **8:** 495 doi:10.3390/foods8100495.

Eidi A, Eidi M, Esmaeili E (2006) Antidiabetic effect of garlic (*Allium sativum* L.) in normal and streptozotocin-induced diabetic rats. *Phytomedicine* 13: 624– 629.

El-Boshy ME, Abdalla OM, Risha A, Moustafa F (2013) Effect of Withania somnifera Extracts on Some Selective Biochemical, Hematological, and Immunological Parameters in Guinea Pigs Experimental Infected with E. coli. *ISRN Vet Sci* Article ID 153427, http://dx.doi.org/10.1155/2013/153427.

Foster CA, Church KS, Poddar M, Van-Uum SH, Spaic T (2017) Licorice-induced hypertension: A case of pseudohyperaldosteronism due to jelly bean ingestion. *PostgradMed* **129**: 3293–3331.

França TGD, Ishikawa LLW, Zorzella-Pezavento SFG, Chiuso-Minicucci F, da Cunha MLRS, Sartori A (2009) Impact of malnutrition on immunity and infection. *J Venom Anim Toxins incl Trop Dis* **15(3)**: 374-390.

Friedman H, Newton C, Klein TW (2003) Microbial Infections, Immunomodulation, and Drugs of Abuse.*Clin Microbiol Rev* **16(2)**: 209–219.

Gautam M, Saha S, Bani S, Kaul A, Mishra S, Patil D, Satti NK, Suri KA, Gairola S, Suresh K, Jadhav S, Qazi GN, Patwardhan B (2009) Immunomodulatory activity of Asparagus racemosus on systemic Th1/Th2 immunity: Implications for immunoadjuvant potential. *J Ethnopharmacol* **121**: 241–247.

Gill MK, Kumar S, Sharma M, Singh TP, Kumar K, Kaur R (2019) Role of Ashwagandha Incorporated Functional Foods for Betterment of Human Health: A Review. *J Agric Eng Food Technol* **6(2)**: 161-165.

Goel A, Singh DK, Kumar S, Bhatia AK (2010) Immunomodulating property of *Ocimum sanctum* by regulating the IL-2 production and its mRNA expression using rat's splenocytes. *Asian Pac J Trop Med* **3(1)**: 8-12.

Goêbiowska-Wawrzyniak M, Markiewicz K, Kozar A, Wanda Karwowska W, Derentowicz P, Siwiñska-Goêbiowska H (2004) Does garlic (aliofil) influence the immune system of children?-A preliminary study. *Pol J Food Nutr Sci* **13(SI 2)**: 29–32.

Gorbalenya AE, Baker SC, Baric RS, de Groot RJ, Drosten C, Gulyaeva AA, Haagmans BL, Lauber C, Leontovich AM, Neuman BW, Penzar D, Perlman S, Poon LLM, Samborskiy D, Sidorov IA, Sola I, Ziebuhr J (2020) Severe acute respiratory syndrome-related coronavirus: the species and its viruses—a statement of the Coronavirus Study Group. bioRxiv, published online Feb 11. DOI:2020.02.07.937862 (preprint).

Halder S, Mehta AK, Mediratta PK (2012) Augmented humoral immune response and decreased cell mediated immunity by *Aloe vera* in rats. *Inflammopharmacology* **20**: 343 346.

Haslberger AG, Jakob U, Hippe B, Karlic H (2020) Mechanisms of selected functional foods against viral infections with a view on COVID-19; Mini review. *Func Food Health Dis* **5(10)**: 195-209.

Hasler CM, Brown AC (2009) Position of the American Dietetic Association: Functional Foods. *J Am Diet Assoc* **109(4)**: 735-746 DOI: 10.1016/j.jada.2009.02.023.

Hemalatha R, Babu KN, Karthik M, Ramesh R, Kumar BD, Kumar PU (2011) Immunomodulatory activity and Th1/Th2 cytokine response of *Ocimum sanctum* in myelosuppressed Swiss Albino mice. *Trends Medical Res* **6(1)**: 23-31 DOI: 10.3923/tmr.2011.23.31.

Huang C, Wang Y, Li X, Ren L, Zhao J, Hu Y, Zhang L, Fan G, Xu J, Gu X, Cheng Z, Yu T, Xia J, Wei Y, Wu W, Xie X, Yin W, Li H, Liu M, Xiao Y, Gao H, Guo L, Xie J, Wang G, Jiang R, Gao Z, Jin Q, Wang J, Cao B (2020) Clinical features of patients infected with 2019 novel coronavirus in Wuhan, China. *Lancet* **395**: 497-506.

Hussain K, Iqbal Z, Abbas R, Khan M, Kashif M (2017) Immunomodulatory Activity of *Glycyrrhiza glabra* Extract against Mixed Eimeria Infection in Chickens. *Int J Agric Biol* **19**: 928-932.

Ilyas N, Sadiq M, Jehangir A (2011) Hepatoprotective effect of garlic (*Allium sativum*) and milk thistle (*Silymarin*) in isoniazid induced hepatotoxicity in rats. *Biomedica* **27**: 166-170.

Indu PC, Awasthi P (2008) Development and Quality Evaluation of Cereal-Legume based Biscuits Enriched with Ashwagandha (*Withania somnifera*) Root Powder. *Int J Appl Agric Sci* **3(1)**: 89-97.

Ishimi Y, Takebayashi J, Tousen Y, Yamauchi J, Fuchino H, Kawano T, Inui T, Yoshimatsu K, Kawahara N (2019)Quality evaluation of health foods containing licorice in the Japanese Market. *Toxicol Rep* **6**: 904–913.

Jayati, Bhatiya AK, Kumar A, Goel A, Gupta S, Rahal A (2013) In vitro antiviral potential of *Ocimum sanctum* leaves extract against New Castle Disease Virus of poultry. *Int J of Microbiol and Immunol Res* **2(7)**: 51-55.

Juntachote T, Berghofer E, Siebenhandl S, Bauer F (2006) The antioxidative properties of Holy basil and Galangal in cooked ground pork. *Meat Sci* **72(3)**: 446-456.

Kahramanoglu I, Chen C, Chen J, Wan C (2019) Chemical Constituents, Antimicrobial Activity, and Food Preservative Characteristics of *Aloe vera* Gel. *Agronomy* **9(12)**: 831 doi:10.3390/agronomy9120831.

Karthikeyan K, Gunasekaran P, Ramamurthy N, Govindasamy S (1999) Anticancer Activity of *Ocimum sanctum*. *Pharm Biol* **37(4)**: 285-290.

Keiss H, Dirsch VM, Hartung T, Haffner T, Trueman L, Auger J, Kahane R, Vollmar AM (2003) Garlic (*Allium sativum* L.) Modulates Cytokine Expression in Lipopolysaccharide-Activated Human Blood Thereby Inhibiting NF-κB Activity. The Journal of Nutrition, **133(7)**: 2171-2175.

Keivan Z, Moloud AZ, Kohzad S, Zahra R (2007) Antiviral activity of *Aloe vera* against herpes simplex virus type 2: An *in vitro* study. *Afr J Biotechnol* **6(15)**: 1770-1773.

Khan TA, Ipshita AH, Mazumdar RM, Abdullah ATM, Islam GMR, Rahman MM (2020) Bioactive polyphenol profiling and in-vitro antioxidant activity of *Tinospora cordifolia* Miers ex Hook F and Thoms : A potential ingredient for functional food development. *Bangladesh J Sci Ind Res* **55(1)**: 23-34.

Kumar S, Rai DC, Singh D (2013) The functional, rheological and sensory attributes of Tulsi (holy basil, *Ocimum sanctum*) extract based herbal ice cream. *The Bioscan* **8(1)**: 77-80.

Kumar V, Dhanjal JK, Kaul SC, Wadhwa R, Sundar D (2020) Withanone and caffeic acid phenethyl ester are predicted to interact with main protease (M^{pro}) of SARS-CoV-2 and inhibit its activity. *J Biomol Struct Dyn* 1-13 https://doi.org/10.1080/07391102. 2020.1772108.

Lachenmeier K, Kuepper U, Musshoff F, MadeaB RH, Lachenmeier DW (2005) Quality control of aloe vera beverages. *Electronic J Environ Agric Food Chem* **4(4)**: 1033–1042.

Lau K, Lee K, Koon C, Cheung CS, Lau C, Ho H, Lee MY, Au SW, Cheng CH, Lau CB, Tsui SK, Wan DC, Waye MM, Wong K, Wong C, Lam CW, Leung P, Fung K (2008) Immunomodulatory and anti-SARS activities of *Houttuynia cordataJ Ethnopharmacol* **118(1)**: 79–85.

Li Z, Le W, Cui Z (2018) A novel therapeutic anticancer property of raw garlic extract via injection but not ingestion. *Cell Death Discov* **4**:108. DOI 10.1038/s41420-018-0122-x.

Lin LT, Hsu WC, Lin CC (2014) Antiviral natural products and herbal medicines. *J Tradit Complement Med* **4**: 24-35.

López-Varela S, González-Gross M, Marcos A (2011) Functional foods and the immune system. *Food Ingredients Brasil* N° 16 www.revista-fi.com22-25.

Luta G, McAnalley BH (2005) *Aloe vera*: chemical composition and methods used to determine its presence in commercial products. *GlycoSci Nutr* **6(4)**: 1–12.

Mehrbod P, Amini E, Tavassoti-Kheiri M (2009) Antiviral Activity of Garlic Extract on Influenza Virus. *Iran J Virol* **3(1)**: 19-23

Menni C, Valdes A, Freydin MB, Ganesh S, El-Sayed Moustafa J, Visconti A, Hysi P, Bowyer RCE, Mangino M, Falchi M, Wolf J, Steves C, Spector T (2020) Loss of smell and taste in combination with other symptoms is a strong predictor of COVID-19 infection. *MedRxiv.*doi:https://doi.org/10.1101/2020.04.05.20048421.

Misra B (2016) Production & Quality assessment of herbal ice lolly with tulsi paste– A healthy and delicious dairy dish.*Int J Appl Res* **2(5)**: 716-719.

Mittal J, Sharma MM, Batra M (2014) Tinospora cordifolia: a multipurpose medicinal plant- A review. *J Med Plants Stud* **2(2)**:32-47.

Mondal S, Varma S, Bamola VD, Naik SN, Mirdha BR, Padhi MM, Mehta N, Mahapatra SC (2011) Double-blinded randomized controlled trial for immunomodulatory effects of Tulsi (*Ocimum sanctum Linn.*) leaf extract on healthy volunteers. *J Ethnopharmacol* **136**: 452-456.

Mousa HA (2017) Prevention and treatment of influenza, influenza-like illness, and common cold by herbal, complementary, and natural therapies. *J Evid Based Complementary Altern Med* **22(1)**: 166-174.

Murthy S, Kanthaiah, Govindaswamy (2014) Hypolipidemic effects of garlic extracts in high fat high cholesterol diet fed rats. *J Evol Med Dent Sci* **3(6)**: 1334-1338.

Narayana NMNK, Fernando WSK, Samaraweera GC (2020) Awareness and Attitude towards Functional Dairy Products among consumers in Western Province of Sri Lanka.*Turkish Journal of Agriculture-Food Science and Technology* **8(6)**: 1308-1314.

Oertelt-Prigione S (2012) The influence of sex and gender on the immune response. *Autoimmun Rev* **11**: A479–A485.

Okwu DE (2004) Phytochemicals and vitamin content of indigenous spices of South Eastern. *Nig J Sust Agric Environ* **6**: 30-37.

Pant M, Ambwani T, Umapathi V (2012) Antiviral activity of Ashwagandha extract on Infectious Bursal Disease Virus Replication. *Indian J Sci Technol* **5(5)**: 2750-2751.

Panyod S, Ho CT, Sheen LY (2020) Dietary therapy and herbal medicine for COVID-19 prevention: A review and perspective. *J Tradit Complement Med* doi: https://doi.org/10.1016/j.jtcme.2020.05.004.

Pavaraj M, Balasubramanian V, Baskaran S, Ramasamy P (2011) Development of Immunity by extract of medicinal plant *Ocimum sanctum* on Common carp (*Cyprinuscarpio* L. *Res J Immunol* **4(1)**:12-18.

Pruett SB (2003) Stress and the immune system-Review. *Pathophysiology* **9**: 133-153.

Ramadan MF (2007) Nutritional value, functional properties and nutraceutical applications of black cumin (*Nigella sativa* L.): an overview. *Int J Food Sci Tech* **42**: 1208–1218.

Rani P, Rani V, Jandu R, Lavanya A, Reena, John J (2020) Effect of Storage on Sensory Acceptability and Oxidative Rancidity of Wheat Biscuits Fortified with *Asparagus racemosus* Root Powder. *Eur J Nutr Food Saf* **12(6)**: 13-22.

Roberfroid MB (2000) Prebiotics and probiotics: are they functional foods? *Am J Clin Nutr* **71**: S1682 – S1687.

Rouf R, Uddin SJ, Sarker DK, Islam MT, Ali ES, JA Shilpi, Nahar L, Tiralongo E, Sarker SD (2020) Antiviral potential of garlic (*Allium sativum*) and its organosulfur compounds: A systematic update of pre-clinical and clinical data. *Trends Food Sci Technol* **104**: 219–234.

Sachan S, Dhama K, Latheef SK, Samad HA, Mariappan AK, Munuswamy P, Singh R, Singh KP, Malik YS, Singh RK (2019) Immunomodulatory Potential of *Tinospora cordifolia* and CpG ODN (TLR21 Agonist) against the VeryVirulent, Infectious Bursal Disease Virus in SPF Chicks *Vaccines* **7(106)** doi:10.3390/vaccines7030106.

Sawant BS, Alawe JR, Rasal KV (2016) Pharmacognostic study of *Glycyrrhiza glabra* Linn- a review. *Inter Ayurv Med J* **4(10)**: 3188-3193.

Scepanovic P, Alanio C, Hammer C, Hodel F, Bergstedt J, Patin E, Thorball CW, Chaturvedi N, Charbit B, Abel L, Quintana-Murci L, Duffy D, Albert ML, Fellay J (2018) Human genetic variants and age are the strongest predictors of humoral immune responses to common pathogens and vaccines. *Genome Med* **10**:59 https://doi.org/10.1186/s 13073-018-0568-8.

Shang A, Cao S, Xu X, Gan R, Tang G, Corke H, Mavumengwana V, Li H (2019) Bioactive Compounds and Biological Functions of Garlic (*Allium sativum* L.). *Foods* **8**: 246-276.

Sharma P, Parmar J, Sharma P, Verma P, Goyal PK (2012) Radiation- induced testicular injury and its amelioration by *T. cordifolia* (An Indian Medicinal plant) extract. *Evid Based Comp Altern Med* 643-647. doi:10.1155/2011/643847

Shevale UL, Mundrawale AS, Yadav SR, Chavan JJ, Jamdade CB, Patil DB (2015) Phytochemical and antimicrobial studies on Asparagus racemosus. *World J Pharm Res* **4(9)**: 1805-1810.

Singh AK, Rai DC, Singh UP, Kumar S (2018) Effect of different variables on physico-chemical properties of Ashwagandha enriched strawberry pulp ice cream. *The Pharm Innov J* **7(4)**: 440-443.

Singh N, Hoette Y, Miller R (2010) Tulsi: The Mother Medicine of Nature. 2nd ed. Lucknow: International Institute of Herbal Medicine. 28 47.

Singh N, Jha A, Chaudhary A, Upadhyay A (2014) Enhancement of the functionality of bread by incorporation of Shatavari (*Asparagus racemosus*). *J Food Sci Technol* **51(9):** 2038-2045

Singhal, T., 2020.A review of coronavirus Disease-2019 (COVID-19).*Indian J. Pediatr.* 87 (April), 281–286.

Sommer AP, Forsterling H, Naber KG (2020) Thymoquinone: shield and sword against SARS-CoV-2. *Precis Nanomed* **3(3):** 541-548.

Strika I, Bašiæ A, Haliloviæ N (2016) Antimicrobial effects of garlic (*Allium sativum* L.) *Glasnik hemièara i tehnologa Bosne i Hercegovina* **47:** 17-20.

Swaminathan C, Santhi M (2019) Phytochemical analysis and antimicrobial activity of roots of Withania somnifera (L.) Dunal. *Int J Chemtech Res* **12(2):** 218-222.

Tapiero H, Townsend DM, Tew KD (2004) Organosulfur compounds from alliaceae in the prevention of human pathologies. *Biomed Pharmacother* **58:** 183-193.

Thakur M, Connellan P, Deseo MA, Morris C, Praznik W, Loeppert R, Dixit VK (2012) Characterization and in vitro immunomodulatory screening of fructo-oligosaccharides of *Asparagus racemosus* Willd. *Int J Biol Macromol* **50:** 77–81.

Tian HY (2020) 2019-nCoV: new challenges from coronavirus. Zhonghua Yu Fang Yi XueZaZhi 54(00): E001-E001. doi: 10.3760/cma.j.issn.0253-9624.2020.0001.

Tiwari R, Chakraborty S, Saminathan M, Dhama K, Singh SV (2014). Ashwagandha (*Withania somnifera*): Role in safeguarding health, immunomodulatory effect, combating infections and therapeutic applications: A review. *J Biol Sci* **14(2):** 77-94.

Tolo FM, Rukunga GM, Muli FW, Njagi EN, Njue W, Kumon K, Kofi- Tsekpo MW (2006) Anti-viral activity of the extracts of a Kenyan medicinal plant *Carissa edulis* against herpes simplex virus. *J Ethnopharmacol* **104(1–2):** 92–99.

Veena N, Arora S, Singh RRB, Katara A, Rastogi S, Rawat KS (2015) Effect of *Asparagus racemosus* (shatavari) extract on physicochemical and functional properties of milk and its interaction with milk proteins. *J Food Sci Technol* **52(2):** 1176–1181. DOI 10.1007/s13197-013-1073-0.

Veena N, Arora S, Kapila S, Singh RRB, Katara A, Pandey MM, Rastogi S, Raeat KS (2014) Immunomodulatory and antioxidative potential of milk fortified with *Asparagus racemosus* (Shatavari). *J Med Plants Stud* **2(6):** 13-19.

Venkatalakshmi P, Vadivel V, Brindha P (2016) Role of phytochemicals as immunomodulatory agents: A review. *Int J Green Pharm* **10(1)**: 1-17.

Verpoorte R., van der Heijden R., Hoopen H. J. and Memelink J. (1999). Metabolic engineering of plant secondary metabolite pathways for the production of fine chemicals. *Biotechnol Lett* **21**: 467-79

Vinaya M, Kudagi BL, Kamdod MA, Swamy M (2017) Bronchodilator activity of *Ocimum sanctum* Linn. (tulsi) in mild and moderate asthmatic patients in comparison with salbutamol: a single blind cross-over study. *Int J Basic Clin Pharmacol* **6**: 511-517.

Viswaroopan D, Arun-Raj GR, Shailaja U, Maurya D, Gawade S, Shivanand P, Jithesh-Raj KT (2015) Preparation of Ashwagandha (*Withania somnifera*L.) Dunal) ghee – A practical approach inspired by traditional knowledge. *Pharm Innov J* **4(4)**: 85-89.

Wadhwa R, Singh R, Gao R, Shah N, Widodo N, Nakamoto T, Ishida Y, Terao K, Kaul SC (2013) Water Extract of Ashwagandha Leaves Has Anticancer Activity: Identification of an Active Component and Its Mechanism of Action. *PLoS ONE* **8(10)**: e77189. doi:10.1371/journal.pone.0077189.

Wang J, Du G, (2020) COVID-19 may transmit through aerosol. *Ir J Med Sci* 1–2 https://doi.org/10.1007/s11845-020-02218-2.

Wang L, Yang R, Yuan B, Liun Y, Liu C (2015) The antiviral and antimicrobial activities of licorice, a widely-used Chinese herb. *Acta Pharm Sin B* http://dx.doi.org/10.1016/j.apsb.2015.05.005.

Wangcharoen W, Morasuk W (2007) Antioxidant capacity and phenolic content of holy basil. *Songklanakarin J Sci Technol* **29**: 1407 15.

WHO (2020) "Immunity passports" in the context of COVID 19. Scientific brief, https://www.who.int/news-room/commentaries/detail/immunity-passports-in-the-context-of-covid-19 (Accessed on September 2nd 2020)

Wu C, Chen X, Cai Y, Xia J, Zhou X, Xu S, Xia J, Zhou X, Xu S, Huang H, Zhang L, Zhou X, Du C, Zhang Y, Song J, Wang S, Chao Y, Yang Z, Xu J, Zhou X, Chen D, Xiong W, Xu L, Zhou F, Jiang J, Bai C, Zheng J, Song Y, (2020) Risk factors associated with acute respiratory distress syndrome and death in patients with coronavirus disease 2019 pneumonia in Wuhan, China. *JAMA Int Med* doi.org/10.1001/jamainternmed.2020.0994.

WWW.Worldometers.info. (2020) COVID-19 coronavirus pandemic. https://www. Worldometers.info/coronavirus/ (Accessed on September 15th, 2020).

Yadav K, Shukla S (2014) Antioxidant activity of green tea and tulsi yogurt. *Trends in Biosciences* **7(21)**: 3465-3467.

Zezelj I, Milosevic J, Stojanovic Z, Ognjanov G (2012) The motivational and informational basis of attitudes toward foods with health claims. *Appetite* **59(3)**: 960-967.

Zhou P, Yang X, Wang X Hu B, Zhang L, Zhang W, Si H, Zhu Y, Li B, Huang C, Chen H, Chen J, Luo Y, Guo H, Jiang R, Liu M, Chen Y, Shen X, Wang X, Zheng X, Zhao K, Chen Q, Deng F, Liu L, Yan B, Zhan F, Wang Y, Xiao G, Shi Z (2020) A pneumonia outbreak associated with a new coronavirus of probable bat origin. *Nature* **579:** 270–273.

Immunity Boosting Functional Foods to Combat COVID-19, Pages: 27–36
Edited by: Apurba Giri

CHAPTER - 2

TULSI-A POTENTIAL IMMUNE BOOSTING FUNCTIONAL FOOD INGREDIENT TO COMBAT COVID-19

Sucheta Sahoo Palai[1] and Apurba Giri[2]*

[1] *State Aided College Teacher, Department of Nutrition,*
E-mail: suchetasahoo12@gmail.com
[2]*Assistant Professor and Head, Department of Nutrition,*
Coordinator, Dept. of Food Processing
E-mail: apurbandri@gmail.com
Mugberia Gangadhar Mahavidyalaya, Bhupatinegar-721425, West Bengal, India
**Corresponding author*

ABSTRACT

Now a days coronavirus is the most discussed topic in everywhere and recent outbreak in the worldwide. At first it was found in Wuhan city, China and then spreaded every corner of the world like a wildfire and finally it becomes pandemic. Coronavirus is basically RNA strands which creates acute respiratory problem. It spreads from human to human which is known as zoonotic transmission. The only way to break the spreading of this chain is social distancing and takes some important precautions like wearing face musk, frequent washing hands by soap etc. Till now there is no vaccine or medicine available, only symptomatic treatment is the only way to cure. Immunity boosting is the most important way to combat COVID-19. Even health experts also revealed that poor immunity is the reason to death by this virus. So, balanced diet, therapeutic diet, adequate sleep, meditation and yoga plays important role to improve immunity power of the human body system. In this regards, Tulsi (*Ociumsanetum*) also plays an important role to boost immunity system as it has many important medicinal properties. This article shows the medicinal importance and characteristics of Tulsi to combat COVID-19 by immunity boosting.

Keywords: Tulsi, Immunity boosting, COVID-19, Pharmaceutical activity, Ayurveda

INTRODUCTION

In the past six months of the current year of 2020, the corona virus has badly affected our daily life, which declared a pandemic on 12 March 2020. This virus acts as a very infectious disease, which mainly causes the acute respiratory syndrome. At first, it was found in the city of Wuhan, China,on 30th January 2020 and gradually became a disaster for the whole world (Patil and Kakde, 2018).

It consists of a group of related RNA viruses that causes illness for the human being. Most people infected by COVID 19 experienced with mild to moderate respiratory disease andit may be recovered without hospitalization. It becomes very critical for the older person and for the person who have any acute disease like diabetes, cardiovascular disease, chronic respiratory disease and cancer. Till now there are lack of proper medicine, vaccine and medical support to combat this virus. Only systematic based treatments are followed to treat a patient (Kulkarni and Adavirao, 2018; Gautam *et al.*, 2020).

COVID 19 spreads through droplets of saliva which discharges from nose and mouth, when an infected person coughs and sneezes. The best way to slow down the transmission is to protect ourself from the virus by using face musk, washing hands with soap and the uses of alcohol based sanitizer and not to frequently touch the face and mouth (Khanal *et al.*, 2020).

Recent study found that immunity is the one of the way to prevent from this infectious disease. Therefore it is highly recommended to boost immunity system to prevent this COVID-19. The ways to improve the immunity system are proper exercise, adequate sleep, meditation, avoid smoking and drinking, and balanced diet (Satuna *et al.*, 2020).

In Ayurveda also there are several plants whichused from ancient times to boost human immune system like tulsi, turmeric, onion, garlic, moringa, amla, giloy, neem, aswagandha, cinnamon, black paper etc.

Tulsi is most recommended traditional medicinal plant which is used for treatment of different kind of diseases which loaded with plenty of different types of antimicrobial, antiseptic properties. It is also used as natural hand sanitizer (Kadian and Parle, 2012). Tulsi also prevents common cold and cough and can strengthen the respiratory system. Tulsi have several pharmacological properties which boost our immunity system to combat COVID-19.

Role of Tulsi to Boost Immune System Against COVID-19

Tulsi is very traditional medicinal plant which has so many therapeutic properties to prevent diarrhea, cough, cold, fever, anxiety, chronic cough, bronchitis etc. (Singh and Majumdar, 1997; Kulkarni and Adavirao, 2018). From the ancient time, Tulsi also considered as a very religious plant in Hindu family and temples. According to Vishnupuran which is a religious book of Hindu, Tulsi is used to serve lord Vishnu to please him (Upadhyay, 2017). Scientific name of Tulsi is *Ocimum sanctum* which belonging in Lamiaceae family. In India Tulsi is available everywhere from Andaman Nicobar to Himalaya (Mohite *et al.*, 2020).

Mainly Tulsi have Two types of Variant (Kulkarni and Adavirao, 2018)

i.   Black Tulsi (Krishna Tulsi)
ii. Green Tulsi (Rama Tulsi)

Table I: Various names of Tulsi in Indian states (Kadian and Parle, 2012)

S.No	State	Name
1.	West Bengal	Tulsi, Kalotulsi, Kural
2.	North-eastern India	Mayangton, Naoshek lei
3.	Assam	Tuloxi, Tulasii
4.	Orissa	Dhalatulasi, Karpura
5.	Andhra Pradesh	Oddhi, Rudrajada
6.	Tamilnadu	Tiruttizhai, Tiviragandam
7.	Karnataka	Karitulasi,Tulasiya
8.	Kerala	Pachcha, Kunnakam
9.	Kashmir	Tulsi, Janglitulsi
10.	Punjab	Tulsi
11.	Maharashtra	Sabja, Tulasa
12.	Gujarat	Sabje, Talasi
13.	Himachal Pradesh	Tulsi, Niyan Posh

Table II: Various names of Tulsi in different countries (Kadian and Parle, 2012)

S. No	Country	Name
1.	Bangladesh	Tulsi, Manjari, Ajaka
2.	Nepal	Bavari phul, Tulsi patta

[Table Contd.

Contd. Table]

S. No	Country	Name
3.	India	Jangli tulsi, Besil, Tulsi
4.	Burma	Laun, Pinzainpinzin
5.	China	Yu heung choi, Loh lahk
6.	Malaya	Kemangi, Selasijantan
7.	Vietnam	Cay hung que, Nhu tia
8.	Thailand	Horapa, Kaphrau
9.	North Africa, Middle East	Vasub,Dohsh,Schadjant
10.	Northeast of Thailand	Phak I tou thai, Saphaa
11.	Netherlands, South Africa	Baziel, Koningskruid
12.	Finland, Sweden, Norway	Basilika
13.	Japan	Bajiru, Kami-meboki
14.	Germany	IndischesBasilikum
15.	France	Herbe royale, Basilic sacre
16.	Sri Lanka	Madurutala, Muduratulla
17.	Spain	Alfabega, Albacar
18.	Cambodia	Mareah proeu, Che tak
19.	Georgia	Rekhani, Rehani
20.	Denmark, Greenland	Basilikum
21.	England	Basilie, Sweet Basil
22.	Iceland	Basilika
23.	Italy	Basilico
24.	Korea	Naruk-pul, Yanggajuk
25.	Bulgaria	Bosilek
26.	Armenia	Shahasbram, Rehan

Chemical Constituent of Tulsi

One special types of volatile oil is concentrated into the leaf of Tulsi, which gives a specific aromatic odor. This oil consists of aldehydes, phenols and terpenes. This plant also contains alkaloids, saponines, glycosides, and tannins. Extracted oil of Tulsi seeds is called fixed oil which mainly formed by fatty acids. Different part of the plant contains different chemical which is shown in Table III(Pandey and Madhuri, 2010).

According to various literatures, an edaphic and geographic factor plays an important role for chemical constituents of Tulsi. In the different part of the world, Tulsi shows some different chemical substances (Joshi *et al.*, 2017).

Table III: Chemical constituent present in *Ocimum Sanctum* (Mondal *et al.,* 2009; Kulkarni and Adavirao, 2018)

Sl. No	Various Parts	Chemical constituents
1.	Seeds	Oleic acid, Stearic acid, Linolenic acid, Palmitic acid, Linoleic acid.
2.	Leaves	Caryphyllene oxide, Broneol, Limonene, Ocimene, Farnesol, Furaldehyde, Farnesene, Cubenol,D-Limonene, Bronyl acetate, Eugenol, α-Pinene, β-Guaiene, Methyl chavicol, Selinene, Camphor, Aromadendene oxide, Germacrene, Farnesol, Phytol, Camphene, n-butylbenzoate, Benzaldehyde, Eicosane, Heptanol, Eucalyptol, Humulene, Oleic acid, Veridifloro, αMyrcene.
3.	Whole Plant	Calcium, Chromium, Zink, Iron, Phosphorus, Copper, Vitamin C, Vitamin A,
4.	Leaves / Areal Parts	Urosolic acid, Vitexin, Apgenin, Circineol, Galuteolin, Circineol, Luteolin, Vallinin, VIlinin acid, caffeic acid, Stigmsterol, Isovitexin, Galic acid, Isorientin, Procatechuic acid, Aesculectin, Molludistin, Orientin.

Morphology

A mature Tulsi plant is about to height of 30-60 cm with simple branched typed aromatic leaves. Leaves are thin types elliptical, up to 5 cm long and clearly show dentate margins. Its purple colour flowers help to enlarge raceme in close whorls of the steam. Fruits are small and seeds are radish yellow. It's a rainy season plant and reaped after few days (Kulkarni and Adavirao, 2018).

Taxonomy

Kingdom: Plantae
  Division: Magnoliophyta
    Class: Magnoliopsida
      Order: Lamiales
        Family: Labiatae
          Genus: Ocimum
            Species: Sanctum

Ayurvedic activity of Tulsi (Kulkarni and Adavirao, 2018)

All parts of Tulsi plants are very much useful in Ayurvedic treatment. At first, all the aerial parts of Tulsi are carefully collected and washed it with clean water.

Then it is cut into small pieces and crashed then with mortar pestle. Final product of Tulsi juice will get after screening the soft and smooth paste by cotton cloth. This juice is useful as Ayurvedic medicine to prevent common colds, headaches, heart disease, stomach disorder etc. Traditionally, Tulsi is used in many forms like dried powder, herbal tea, fresh leaf with honey etc. (Chattopadhyay, 1993; Agrawal *et al.,* 1996). Different parts of Tulsi are used for different medicinal purpose are shown in Table IV.

Table IV: Different parts of Tulsi used for various therapeutic activity (Kulkarni and Adavirao, 2018)

Sl. No	Parts used for extraction	Therapeutic activity
1.	Whole plant (dried)	Anti-stress
2.	Leaves	Anti-inflammatory
3.	Leaves	Anti-fungal
4.	Leaves	Anti-fertility
5.	Whole plant (aerial)	Hepatoprotective
6.	Leaves	Anti-diabetic
7.	Leaves	Anti-ulcer
8.	Leaves	Anti-microbial
9.	Leaves	Anti-psychotic
10.	Root	Anti-cancer

Pharmaceutical activity

Presence of various type of chemical compound in Tulsi which have different kind of pharmaceutical and biological activity that are discussed as follows (Khanal *et al.,* 2020).

1. **Anti-inflammatory activity:** Singh and Majumdar (1997) opined that fixed oil of *O. Sanctum* act as an anti-inflammatory agent due to presence linolenic acid. It also act as an inhibitor of lipoxygenase and cyclooxygenase pathways of arachidonate metabolism.

2. **Anti-stress activity:** Jyoti*et al.* (2007) suggested that *O. Sactum* leaves has the potentiality to decrease the stress. They examine on experimentally induced oxidative stress rabbits and they observed that these leaves have anti-stress activity (Jyoti *et al.,* 2007).

3. **Anti-diabetic activity:** Bihari *et al.* (2011) found that the leaf extract of *O. Sanctum* have the ability to show anti-diabetic activity and it is highly comparable with the standard drugs of glibenclamide. In comparision with

other medicine and different species of Oscimum, methanolic extract of *O. Sactum*have better anti-diabetic function.

4. **Anti-fungal activity:** Anti-fungal activity of *O. Sanctum* was verified against dermatophytes. Anti-fungal activity of linalool and methyl chavicol present in *Ocimum sanctum* have the potential effect on azole-resistant strains and candida (Balakumar *et al.*, 2011).

5. **Anti-fertility activity:** Sperm count and motility of sperm are decreased by *O. Sanctum*. Researchers reported that this effect is mainly due to deprivation of androgen by its anti-androgenic character. These leaves act as a contraceptive compound (Gupta *et al.*, 2002).

6. **Anti-bacterial activity:** Mishra and Mishra (2011) evaluated the effect of anti-bacterial character *O. Sanctum* leaves by experimenting on gram negative and gram positive bacteria. Oil extracted from these leaves added with chloroform and alcohol shows anti-bacterial activity *against P. aeruginosa, S. aureus, E. coli*. Extract also have the same effect against gram negative and gram positive bacteria (Poonam and Sanjay, 2011)

7. **Anticancer activity:** Monga *et al.* (2011) showed that alcoholic extract of the leaves have anti-melanoma activity. These leave extract significantly reduce the tumor volume and increase survival rate (Pandey, 2009; Madhuri and Pandey, 2010).

8. **Anticoagulant activity:** *Ocimum sanctum* oil has the ability to increase blood clotting time due to anti-aggregatory function of extract on platelets. The response is also similar with aspirin (Singh *et al.*, 2001).

9. **Anticataleptic activity:** Alcoholic extract of the *Ocimum sanctum* leaf have anticataleptic function and reduce the cataleptic rate(Kadian and Parle, 2012).

10. **Antiemetic activity:** Tulsi leaves was also used to check vomiting and antiemetic action (Kumar *et al.*, 2011).

11. **Antihelminthic activity:** Asha*et al.* (2001) evaluated the potential effect of essential oil and eugenol obtained from *Ocimum sanctum* leaves on the antihelminthic activity by Caenorhabditis elegans model.

12. **Anti-plasmodial activity:** Inbaneson *et al.* (2012) showed that *Ocimum sanctum* leaf extract contain saponins, triterpenoids, tannins, flavonoids, glycosides, proteins, phenols, steroids which have the important role in anti-plasmodial activity.

13. **Anti-ulcer activity:** Presence of lipoxygenase inhibitory and antisecretory effects, it showed important role in anti-ulcer activity in rats (Singh *et al.*, 2001).

Ways for consumption of Tulsi

Tulsi has many therapeutic properties to increase immunity boosting potential during COVID-19 period. We can use various parts of Tulsi and the different ways of consumption are discussed by points.

i. Tulsi leaves are used with honey and ghee.

ii. Tulsi leaves can be used in hot water as herbal Tulsi tea.

iii. Dried Tulsi powder with lukewarm water, lemon and honey can be used as morning drink.

iv. Tulsi leaves and whole plant used as an Ayushkwath.

v. Extracted essential oil from Tulsi used in different types of medicine.

CONCLUSION

Now a day COVID-19 creates too much panic in our mind all over the world. There are no medicine, no vaccine, even not any particular treatment. Only way to prevent this situation is social distancing, covering face mask, washing hands frequently and most importantly immunity boosting to our body. So that body can fight against coronavirus. In this perspective Tulsi plays important role which has not only immunity boosting property but also have so many therapeutic properties. Tulsi also called Queen of herb because of its tremendous pharmacological properties. From the ancient time, Tulsi used by human in various form to cure anti-inflammatory, anti-diabetic, anti-stress, anti-fungal and so many.

REFERENCES

Agrawal P, Rai V, Singh RB (1996) Randomized placebo-controlled, single blind trial of holy basil leaves in patients with noninsulin-dependent diabetes mellitus. *Int J Clin Pharm Th* **34(9):** 406–409.

Patil A, Kakde M (2018) Medicinal plant as a natural immunity booster for COVID19- A review. *Indian J Integr Med* **2(2):** 187–194.

Asha MK (2001) Anthelmintic activity of essential oil of *Ocimum sanctum* and eugenol. *Fitoterapia* **72(6):** 669–670.

Balakumar S (2011) Antifungal activity of *Ocimum sanctum* Linn.(Lamiaceae) on clinically isolated dermatophytic fungi. *As Pa J Trop Med* **4(8):** 654–657.

Bihari CG, Behera M, Panda SK, Tripathy SK (2011) Phytochemical investigation & evaluation for antidiabetic activity of leafy extracts of various Ocimum (Tulsi) species by alloxan induced diabetic model. *J Pharm Res* **4(1):** 28–29.

Chattopadhyay RR (1993) Hypoglycemic effect of Ocimum sanctum leaf extract in normal and streptozotocin diabetic rats. *Indian J ExpBiol* **31(11):** 891–893.

Gautam S (2020) Immunity against COVID-19: Potential role of AyushKwath. *J Aim*doi: 10.1016/j.jaim.2020.08.003.

Gupta SK, Prakash J, Srivastava S (2002) Validation of traditional claim of Tulsi, *Ocimum sanctum* Linn.as a medicinal plant. *Indian J Biotechnol* **40(7):** 765–773.

Inbaneson SJ, Sundaram R, Suganthi P (2012) In vitro antiplasmodial effect of ethanolic extracts of traditional medicinal plant Ocimum species against Plasmodium falciparum. *Asian Pac J Trop Med* **5(2):** 103–106.

Joshi RK, Setzer WN, Silva JK (2017) Phytoconstituents, traditional medicinal uses and bioactivities of Tulsi (*Ocimum sanctum* Linn.): A review. *Am J Essent Oil Nat Prod* **5(1):** 18–21.

Jyoti S, Satendra S, Sushma S, Anjana T, Shashi S (2007) Antistressor activity of Ocimum sanctum (Tulsi) against experimentally induced oxidative stress in rabbits. *Method Find Exp Clin* **29(6):** 411–416.

Kadian R, Parle M (2012) Therapeutic potential and phytopharmacology of tulsi. *Int J Pharm Life Sci* **3(7):** 1858–1867.

Khanal P (2020) Network pharmacology of AYUSH recommended immune-boosting medicinal plants against COVID-19: 1–12. *Research Sqr* doi:10.21203/rs.3.rs-31776/v1

Kumar V (2011) Pharmacological Review on *Ocimum sanctum* Linnaeus/ : A Queen of herbs. *J Pharm Sci* **4(2):** 366–368.

Kulkarni KV, Adavirao BV (2018) A review on: Indian traditional shrub Tulsi (Ocimum sanctum): the unique medicinal plant. *J Med Plant Stud* **6(2):** 106-110.

Kushwah P, Kayande N, Mohite B (2020) Corona virus (COVID-19): An Ayurvedic approach (Possible role of Tulsi). *Int J Pharmacogn Phytochem* **9(2):** 2361–2362.

Madhuri S, Pandey G (2010) Effect of proimmu, a herbal drug on estrogen caused uterine and ovarian cytotoxicity. *Biomed* **5(1):** 57–62.

Mishra P, Mishra S (2011) Study of Antibacterial Activity of Ocimum sanctum Extract Against Gram Positive and Gram Negative Bacteria. *Am J Food Technol* **6:** 336-341.

Monga J, Sharma M, Tailor N, Ganesh N (2011) Antimelanoma and radioprotective activity of alcoholic aqueous extract of different species of Ocimum in C(57)BL mice. *Pharm Biol* **49(4):** 428–436.

Mondal S, Mirdha BR, Mahapatra SC (2009) The science behind sacredness of Tulsi (*Ocimum sanctum*Linn.). *J Physiol Pharmacol* **53(4):** 291–306.

Pandey G (2009) An overview on certain anticancer natural products. *J Pharm Res* **2(12):** 1799–1803.

Pandey G, Madhuri S (2010) Pharmacological activities of *Ocimum sanctum* (Tulsi): A review. *Int J Pharm Sci Rev Res* **5(1):** 61–66.

Poonam M, Sanjay M (2011) Study of antibacterial activity of Ocimum sanctum extract against gram positive and gram negative bacteria. *Am J Food Technol* **6:** 336–341.

Satuna RK, Negi A, Satuna R (2020) Intuitive Vision and Indigenous Immunity Boosting approaches for COVID19: From the Literature of PanditShriram Sharma Acharya. *Dev Sans Interdiscip Int J* **16:** 01–15.

Singh S, Majumdar DK (1997) Evaluation of antiinflammatory activity of fatty acids of *Ocimum sanctum* fixed oil. *Indian J Exp Biol* **35(4):** 380–383.

Singh S, Rehan HM, Majumdar, DK (2001) Effect of Ocimum sanctum fixed oil on blood pressure, blood clotting time and pentobarbitone-induced sleeping time. *J Ethnopharmacol* **78(2–3):** 139—143.

Upadhyay RK (2017) Tulsi: A holy plant with high medicinal and therapeutic value. *Int J Green Pharm* **11(1):** S1–S12.

Venkatrao AB, Vilas KK (2018) A review on: Indian traditional shrub Tulsi (*Ocimum sanctum*): The unique medicinal plant. *J Med Plants Stud* **6(2):** 106–110.

Immunity Boosting Functional Foods to Combat COVID-19, Pages: 37–46
Edited by: Apurba Giri

CHAPTER-3

POTENTIAL USE OF CURCUMIN TO COMBAT COVID-19

Monalisa Roy[1] and Apurba Giri[2*]

[1]*Assistant Professor, Dept. of Food Processing,*
E-mail: monalisaroy1997@gmail.com
[2]*Assistant Professor and Head, Dept. of Nutrition,*
Coordinator, Dept. of Food Processing,
E-mail: apurbandri@gmail.com
Mugberia Gangadhar Mahavidyalaya, Bhupatinagar,
Purba Medinipur-721425, West Bengal, India
*Corresponding author

ABSTRACT

In recent time's novel corona virus (CoV) have created an emergency throughout the world. It periodic transmission of CoV introduces the current risk to human health and global economy. Since no fruitful treatment for this infection has not introduced yet. Present review study is carried out to deliver the health promoting effect of curcumin including its activity as an antiviral agent. Curcumin, the pigment present in turmeric has tremendously studied by the researcher from various aspects. It can be extracted from turmeric by several processes. The corona virus provoke pneumonia is connected with unreasonable inflammatory response. In the lung the inflammatory response is known as cytokine storms. Acute Lung Injury (ALI), and Pulmonary oedema are the consequences of the cytokine storms. Curcumin have antiviral, anti-inflametory activity andantioxidant properties that also used as a therapy of ALI/ acute respiretory distress syndrome (ARDS). Due to lower water solubility and biological availability researchers are developing various biocompatible formulations like liposome, cellulose, non emulsionetc. As a nutritional supplement curcumin with vitamin c and zinc could be a powerful weapon against corona virus infection. However, to prove the fact a large amount of clinical trials is required.

Keywords: Curcumin, CoV, anti-inflammatory, cytokine storms, acute lung injury, drug delivery

INTRODUCTION

COVID-19 has come out as epidemic in China (December, 2019) and spread over the globe, creates a pandemic. Severe acute respiratory syndrome coronavirus 2 (SARS-COV-2) is a novel corona virus and mainly responsible for this disease. The virus is of coronaviridae family. Through respiratory droplets the single stranded positive sense RNA viruses transmitted to humans. The infected patient with SARS COVID, experiences acute respiratory irritation due to raised levels of pro-inflamatorycytokines. When a person is infected through food, several other clinical problems also occur like diarrhea (Zhang et al., 2020; Jean et al., 2020; Das et al., 2020). There is no precise antiviral therapy accessible to combat COVID-19 till. Clinical studies suggested that some conditions therapy to treat the COVID patient which include (antiviral agent, anti-inflammatory agent, and antibiotics (Jean et al., 2020) including the drug hydroxyl-chloroquinone that are generally used in developing countries. In the situation of supportive and preventive therapy polyphenolic compound having mechanism, were extracted from natural products. The antiviral property hasthe ability to target the virus host by specific interactions, viral entry replication. By depending on this fin dings in line the natural compound curcumin has been widely recognized by the antiviral activity. From the roots of curcuma longa the natural polyphenol compound curcumin is extracted and it exhibits a wide range a medicinal and therapeutic properties like antimicrobial, antioxidant, anti-inflammatory, anti-proliferative, cardio protective, and neuro-protective effects. The yellow pigment curcumin extracted from turmeric is widely used in our traditional Indian herbal medicines for the treatment of many disease related inflammation and infection for a longer period (Pang et al., 2015). It is studied that curcumin exhibits antiviral effects, against several viruses like HIV, HPV,HSV-2, influenza virus, zika virus, adenovirus, hepatitis Virus (Praditya et al., 2019; Das et al., 2020). Recently it has been investigated that similar original SARS COV2 also occupy human host by target the Angiotensin Converting Enzyme -2 (ACE-2) membrane receptor, it is an entrance of corona virus. Depending on the existing evidences of therapeutic properties of curcumin, it can be proposed that curcumin can acts as a potential inhibitory agent. It can block the host viral interaction at an entrance site in humans (Jean et al., 2020) and can acts as an attenuator via adjusting the pro inflammatory effects of Angiotensin – II AI receptor signaling pathways by reducing the respiratory distress in the therapy of COVID-19. Curcumin with zinc and vitamin C have showed favorable results to boost the natural immunity. The nutritional supplement also acts as a protective defense against the CoV infection in many patients who are under treatment in Indian settings. It is also studied that using the Nano emulsion system many pharmalogical formulation have been developed and proved the bioavailability, increased solubility with enhanced antihypertensive effect (Rachmawati *et al.*, 2016).

Source of Curcumin

Turmaric is the indigenous of tropical South Asia. To prosper properly it needs a noticeable amount of rainfall annually and temperatures between $25\text{-}30^R{}^"C$. As a dried stem of an herbaceous plant, it is closely related to ginger. The spice turmeric is generally comes from the root *Curcumalonga, L.* that is a member of ginger family. In this carcuma species some major curcuminoids, demethoxycurcumin, curcumin and bisdemethoxycurcumin occurs naturally. Sometime turmeric is also called the 'Indian Saffron' because of its yellow color. Curcumin, the bright yellow pigment, present in turmeric,isused for natural food coloring agent. Due to its various medicinal properties, preservative effect of the spice has been used for an age (Rachmawati *et al.*, 2016).

The yellow color compound curcumin is mainly extracted from the stem of turmeric. The bioactive effect of turmeric may be due the action of curcumin. Recent studies show that curcumin is responsible for the inhibitory effect of carcinogenesis and angiogenesis. It has many medicinal attributes like antioxidant, anti-inflammatory, antifungal, antibacterial, antiviral, and chemo preventive actions of cancer.

Curcumin the Antiviral Agent

Various studies also published that curcumin can prevent the viral infection process through several mechanisms as like as inhibition of gene expression by obstruct the virus entrance, direct select to viral protein inhibition of particle production, through budding and replication process. (Wen *et al.*, 2007; Basu*et al.*, 2013; Ou *et al.*, 2013; Du *et al.*, 2017; Kolandaivel and Kannan, 2017; Yang *et al.*, 2017; Dai *et al.*, 2018; Praditya *et al.*, 2019). Recent studies have showed that, curcumin helps to prevent Respiratory Syndrome Virus (RSV) by obstruct the attachment to host cells (Yang *et al.*, 2017). The study also showed that curcumin helps to prevent the replication of respiratory syndrome virus in human nasal epithelial cells. Another study also shown that curcuma helps to prevent Procein Reproductive and Respiratory Syndrome Virus (PRRSV). Possibly this prevention was held by the disruption of the liquidity of viral envelop (Du *et al.*, 2017). The obstruction of virus infection by the inhibition of PRRSV- mediated cell function, internalization of virus and uncoading was done by curcumin also (Du *et al.*, 2017).

Century of the world has witness of various pandemic outbreaks that main causes are several subtypes of H5N1, H1V1, IAV, H3N2 and H2N2.Various studies also reported that curcumin and its derived from have the ability to bind hemaglutnin (HA). Influenza virus contain a vital capsid glycoprotein which interferes in virus attachment (Kannan and Kolandaivel, 2017). Curcumin can interact with hemaglutinin and disturbs the membrane structure integrity. Due to that a blockage occurs in the binding site of virus and host cell and thus prevents the IAV entry. Curcumin has the capability to inactivate different strains of IAV and can puzzle their adsorption and obstruct there replication cells infected with IAV (Ou*et al.*, 2013). The mechanism behind this said activity is the activation of NF-E2 related factor2 (NRF2) hemoxygenase-1(HO-1) axis, a classical anti-oxidative and anti-inflammatory signaling which shows the antiviral activity (Dai *et al.*, 2018). Further study reveals that curcumin has a potential role in SARS –CoV(Wen *et al.*, 2007).

Curcumin Against Corona Virus

Due to high rate of mortality of corona virus infection has received a noticeable attention for the last two decades. The evidence from current research reveals that the cytokine storm performsan important role in the growth and development of fatal pneumonia. The patient who experienced SARS-CoV infection from them many illustrates AI and ARDS. The rate of death was greater than 10% (Peiris *et al.*, 2004). The syndrome is also similar to MERS-CoV2 infection. Mortality rate is high in fatal pneumonia due to hyper activation of immune cells in lung (Channappanavar and Perlman, 2017). For the CoV infection one of the essential strategy is to target the cytokine storm. In several clinical trials it has been showed that glucocorticoids also used for the therapy of viral pneumonia. Glucocorticoids have some therapeutic features also. But, it has been studied that a high dosage of glucocorticoids can create a various number of side effects like osteoporosis. A little dosage of glucocorticoids can cause development of lung injury (Buchman, 2001). Similarly different clinical investigation is carried out and the result indicates that the importance of seeking alternative agents having greater effectiveness and lower toxicity are increasing rapidly.

For the treatment of lung index and survival rate curcumin has a potential effect. It reduce the sharpness of viral pneumonia by inhibit the generation of inflammatory cytokines and signaling of NAkb in macrophages. Curcumin has significant role in the activation of Nrf2 in association with reduce oxidative stress and inhibition of TRL2/4, $_p$38/jnk, MAPK and response of NF-›B in feedback to the infection of IAV, and due to the fact improved pneumonia (Dai *et al.*, 2018).

Different studies also reported that curcumin helps to prevention of various disease and it has beneficial role on human health (DiSilvestro *et al.*, 2012; Zhu *et al.*, 2019). Consumption of little amount of curcumin (80mg/day) generates several health benefit attributes like indirect and direct action of antioxidant (DiSilvestro *et al.*, 2012). Depending on the existing evidences from several animal studies it can be concluded that development of severe pneumonia can be prevented by curcumin. In early phase of acute lung injury (ALI), curcumin at the level of 5mg/kg/day helps to defeat structural remodeling of lungs and paraquat induced inflammation in lungs (Tyagi *et al.*, 2016). Pre-administration curcumin helps to decrease mortality rate (Lai *et al.*, 2020). Surprisingly, the mortality rate also decreases by pre-administration with curcumin (Lai *et al.*, 2020). All the existing evidence reports that curcumin has both therapeutic and prophylactic effects on virus induced pneumonia and mortality. However, at present no data is available on the human trials, link between corona virus and curcumin. Depending on its therapeutic and preventive application curcumin could be advised as a medicinal agent for the treatment of coronavirus infection.

Immunomedulatory Effect of Curcumin

Curcumin has tremendous use against aneroxia, cough, hepatic disorder, diabetic wounds, biliary disorder, cryozea and rheumatism. In various experimental animal study and *in vivo* analysis the anti-inflammatory and antioxidant activity of curcumin is widely studied. Curcumin raises titer, the circulating antibody and increases the count of total white blood cell against sheep red blood cells (SRBC). The yellow pigment has also increased the cells forms plaque in the mice spleen. The animals which are treated by curcumin also showed a significant increasing level of phagocytic activity of macrophages. A large number of evidence has confirmed that curcumin acts as an anti-cancers agent and perform its function by regulating several targets in tumor cells. Curcumin promotes the apoptosis of tumor cell through targeting before phosphorylation of I_KB_α inhibits $NF_{-K}B$ activation production of reactive oxygen species. Curcumin also prevents the initiation of cancer mediated tumor in association with ROS, reactive nitrogen species,NF-›B,(NF-E2)-related factor 2,heme oxygenase-1, glutathione reductase, glutathione S-transferase. It is reported that in *in vivo* analysis curcumin has the ability to modulate the immune cell profile of intestine. As a result generation of intestinal tumors cell gets inhibited.

Inhibition of neutrophil activation, inhibition of Mixed Lymphocyte Reaction (MLR), smooth muscle proliferation and suppression of blood monolayer cells proliferation was done by curcumin in *in vitro* analysis (Thangapazham, 2006).

Various researches reported that curcumin regulates the profile of cytokine. The main role in immune system was played by interleukin (IL-12). Interleukin drives the immune response towards the Th1 typeswhich is identified by lower IL4 production and higher interferon γ.

Way of delivery

Curcumin is insoluble in water and the bioavailability of this pigment is very low and that's why researchers are searching and developing new formulation depending on biocompatible organic compounds like cellulose, lyposome, polyethylene glycols, hydrogel, corn oil, etc (Li *et al.,* 2005; Kunwar *et al.,* 2006; Prasad *et al.,* 2014). Supramolecular assembles of the pigment with cucurbyturyl and cyclodextrin have been studied also. This system makes the curcumin biologically available and increases its solubility to water. By the hydrophobic interactions, curcumin gets entrapped to the hydrophilic pockets in this system. Thus the solubility increases. Surprisingly the curcumin fluroscenseis increased when get soluble in any of this system. It is studied that the bioavailability of curcumin in cells is increased best in liposomal form (Kunwar *et al.,* 2006). In market the liposomal based product of curcumin is marketed for various dietary applications. For improvement of activity, delivery and specificity researchers are preparing formulations of curcumin that can bound to oxide nanoparticles and novel metals. This kind of formulations also increased anticancer activity of curcumin. In case of low water soluble drugs, mesoporous silica nanoparticles are significantly used for improvement of its bioavailability (Chin *et al.,* 2009; Jin *et al.,* 2011; Dinda *et al.,* 2012; Yan *et al.,* 2012; Jin *et al.,* 2012; Patra *et al.,* 2013; Gangwar*et al.,* 2013; Singh *et al.,* 2014; Ma'mani*et al.,* 2014). Due to their larger surface area, high pore volume, nanoporus structure MSN can show their action nicely. They are biocompatible in nature and exhibit many biomedical function. Recently gold nano particles based formulation has been studied. For the treatment of cancer, drug delivery, diagnosis of cancer gold nanoparticles showed its importance in medicine and biology (Singh *et al.,* 2013; Sreelakshmi *et al.,* 2013; Sindhu *et al.,* 2014). Singh *et al.,* (2013) invented a conjugate as of gold and curcumin by mixing the gold and curcumin at very high temperature and it showed high antioxidant activity in the assay of DPPH. Another study reported that curcumin was treated with at first hyaluronic acid and after that gold salt and it showed greater cytotoxicity than the pure curcumin in cancer cells (Sreelakshmi *et al.,* 2013). Curcumin had tremendous antimicrobial activity and that was the reason it was conjugated with silver and cobalt nanoparticles (Gangwar *et al.,* 2012; Ravindra *et al.,* 2014). It was also studied that pharmalogical formulation of nanoemulsion system containing curcumin showed higher level of bioavailability and solubility with enhancement of antihypertensive effect (Ravindra *et al.*, 2014).

CONCLUSION

Our Mother- Nature has gifted us this very special molecule (e.g. curcumin) to safeguard human from various chronic disease. The molecule present in turmeric in a very stable natural form. However in addition with vitamin C and zinc curcumin can exhibit encouraging result that can increase the natural immunity power and protective resistance against the infection of CoV and the incident is observed in several hospitalized patient in all over India. Depending on the previous studies of curcumin's biological properties, system of drug delivery, it could be treated as an active molecule against SARS CoV2 infection. Yet a larger investigation of clinical trials is required to understand the importance of curcumin for the treatment of COVID-19.

REFERENCES

Basu P, Dutta S, Begum R, Mittal S, Dutta PD, Bharti AC, Panda CK, Biswas J, Dey B, Talwar GP, Das BC (2013) Clearance of cervical human papillomavirus infection by topical application of curcumin and curcumin containing polyherbal cream: a phase II randomized controlled study. *Asian Pac J Cancer Prev* **14(10):** 5753-9.

Basu P, Dutta S, Begum R, Mittal S, Dutta PD, Bharti AC, Panda CK, Biswas J, Dey B, Talwar GP, Das BC (2013) Clearance of cervical human papillomavirus infection by topical application of curcumin and curcumin containing polyherbal cream: a phase II randomized controlled study. *Asian Pac J Cancer Prev* **14(10):** 5753-9.

Buchman AL (2001) Side effects of corticosteroid therapy.*J ClinGastroenterol* **33(4):** 289-94.

Channappanavar R, Perlman S (2017) Pathogenic human coronavirus infections: causes and consequences of cytokine storm and immunopathology.Springer Berlin Heidelberg **39(5):** 529-539.

Chin SF, Iyer KS, Saunders M, Pierre TG, Buckley C, Paskevicius M, Raston CL (2009) Encapsulation and sustained release of curcumin using superparamagnetic silica reservoirs. *Chem* **15:** 5661–5665.

Dai J, Gu L, Su Y, Wang Q, Zhao Y, Chen X, Deng H, Li W, Wang G, Li K (2018) Inhibition of curcumin on influenza A virus infection and influenzal pneumonia via oxidative stress, TLR2/4, p38/JNK MAPK and NF-κB pathways. *Int Immunopharmacol* **54**:177-87.

Das S, Sarmah S, Lyndem S, Singha Roy A (2020) An investigation into the identification of potential inhibitors of SARS-CoV-2 main protease using molecular docking study. *J Biomol Struct Dyn* 1-8.doi.org/10.1080/07391102.2020.1763201.

Dinda AK, Prashant CK, NaqviSS, Unnithan J, Samim M, Maitra A (2012)Curcumin loaded organically modified silica (ORMOSIL) nanoparticle; A novel agent for cancer therapy. *IntJ Nanotechnol* **9(10-12):** 862–871.

DiSilvestro RA, Joseph E, Zhao S, Bomser J (2012) Diverse effects of a low dose supplement of lipidated curcumin in healthy middle aged people. *Nutr J* **11(1):** 79.

Du T, Shi Y, Xiao S, Li N, Zhao Q, Zhang A, Nan Y, Mu Y, Sun Y, Wu C, Zhang H (2017) Curcumin is a promising inhibitor of genotype 2 porcine reproductive and respiratory syndrome virus infection. *BMC Vet Res* **13(1):**1-9.

Gangwar RK, Tomar GB, Dhumale VA, Zinjarde S, Sharma RB, Datar S (2013) Curcumin conjugated silica nanoparticles for improving bioavailability and its anticancer applications. *J Agric Food Chem* **61(40):** 9632–9637.

Jean SS, Lee PI, Hsueh PR (2020) Treatment options for COVID-19: The reality and challenges. *J Microbiol Immuno* **53(3):**436-443.

Jin D, Lee JH, Seo ML, Jaworski J, Jung JH (2012) Controlled drug delivery from mesoporoussili causing a pH response release. *New J Chem* **36(8):** 1616–1620.

Jin D, Park KW, Lee JH, Song K, Kim JG, Seo ML, Jung JH (2011) The selective immobilization of curcumin onto the internal surface of mesoporous hollow silica particles by covalent bonding and its controlled release. *J Mater Chem* **21(11):** 3641–3645.

Kale SN, Datar S (2012) Conjugation of curcumin with PVP capped gold nanoparticles for improving bioavailability. *Mater Sci Eng* **32(8):** 2659–2663.

Kannan S, Kolandaivel P (2017) Antiviral potential of natural compounds against influenza virus hemagglutinin. *Comput Biol Chem* **71:** 207-218.

Kunwar A, Barik A, Pandey R, Priyadarsini KI (2006) Transport of liposomal and albumin loadedcurcumin to living cells: An absorption and fluorescence spectroscopic study. *BBA* **1760(10):** 1513–1520.

Li L, Braiteh FS, Kurzrock R (2005) Liposome-encapsulated curcumin: *in vitro* and *in vivo* effects on proliferation, apoptosis, signaling, and angiogenesis. *Cancer Interdis Int J Am Cancer Soc* **104(6):** 1322–1331.

Ma'mani L, Nikzad S, Kheiri-Manjili H, al-Musawi S, Saeedi M, Askarlou S, Foroumadi A, Shafiee A (2014)Curcumin-loaded guanidine functionalized PEGylatedI3ad mesoporous silica nanoparticles KIT-6:Practical strategy for the breast cancer therapy.*EurJMed Chem* **83:** 646–654.

Ou JL, Mizushina Y, Wang SY, Chuang DY, Nadar M, Hsu WL (2013) Structure–activity relationship analysis of curcumin analogues on anti-influenza virus activity. *FEBS J* **280(22):** 5829–5840.

Pang XF, Zhang LH, Bai F, Wang NP, Garner RE, McKallip RJ, Zhao ZQ(2015) Attenuation of myocardial fibrosis with curcumin is mediated by modulating expression of angiotensin II AT1/AT2 receptors and ACE2 in rats. *Drug Des Dev Ther* **9:** 6043-6054.

Patra D, Sleem FF (2013) A new method for pH triggered curcumin release by applying poly(l-lysine) mediated nanoparticle-congregation. *Anal Chim Acta* **795:** 60–68.

Peiris JSM, Guan Y, Yuen K (2004) Severe acute respiratory syndrome. *Nat Med* **10(12):** S88-S97.

Praditya D, Kirchhoff L, Brüning J, Rachmawati H, Steinmann J, Steinmann E (2019) Anti-infective properties of the golden spice curcumin. *Front Microbiol* **10:** 912.

Prasad S, Tyagi AK, Aggarwal BB (2014)Recent developments in delivery, bioavailability, absorption and metabolism of curcumin: The golden pigment from golden spice. *Cancer Res Treat* **46(1):** 2–18.

Rachmawati H, Soraya IS, Kurniati NS, Rahma A (2016) In vitro study on antihypertensive and antihypercholesterolemic effects of a curcumin nanoemulsion. *Sci Phar.* **84(1):**131–140.

Ravindra S, Mulaba-Bafubiandi AF, Rajinikanth V, Varaprasad K, Reddy NN, Raju KM (2012) Development and characterization of curcumin loaded silver nanoparticle hydrogels for antibacterial and drug delivery applications. *J Inorg Organomet Polym Mate* **22(6):** 1254-1262.

Sindhu K, Rajaram A, Sreeram KJ, Rajaram R (2014)Curcumin conjugated gold nanoparticle synthesis and its bioavailability. *RSC Adv* **4(4):** 1808–1814.

Singh DK, Jagannathan R, Khandelwal P, Abraham PM, Poddar P(2013) In situsynthesis and surface functionalization of gold nanoparticles with curcumin and their antioxidant properties: An experimental and density functional theory investigation. *Nanoscale* **5(5):** 1882–1893.

Singh SP, Sharma M, Gupta PK(2014) Enhancement of phototoxicity of curcumin in human oral cancer cells using silica nanoparticles as delivery vehicle. *Lasers Med Sci* **29(2):** 645–652.

Sreelakshmi C, Goel N, Datta KK, Addlagatta A, Ummanni R, Reddy BV (2013) Green synthesis of curcumin capped gold nanoparticles and evaluation of their cytotoxicity. *Nanosci Nanotechnol* **5(12):** 1258–1265.

Thangapazham RL, Sharma A, Maheshwari RK (2006) Multiple molecular targets in cancer chemoprevention by curcumin. *AAPS J* **8(3):** E443-E449.

Wen CC, Kuo YH, Jan JT, Liang PH, Wang SY, Liu HG, Lee CK, Chang ST, Kuo CJ, Lee SS, Hou CC (2007) Specific plant terpenoids and lignoids possess potent antiviral activities against severe acute respiratory syndrome coronavirus. *J Med Chem* **50(17):** 4087-4095.

Yan H, Teh C, Sreejith S, Zhu L, Kwok A, Fang W, Ma X, Nguyen KT, Korzh V, Zhao Y (2012) Functional mesoporous silica nanoparticles for photothermal-controlled drug delivery. *Angew Chem Int* **51(33):** 8373–8377.

Yang XX, Li CM, Li YF, Wang J, Huang CZ (2017) Synergistic antiviral effect of curcumin functionalized graphene oxide against respiratory syncytial virus infection. *Nanoscale* **9(41):** 16086-16092.

Zhang H, Penninger JM, Li Y, Zhong N, Slutsky AS (2020) Angiotensin-converting enzyme 2 (ACE2) as a SARS-CoV-2 receptor: molecular mechanisms and potential therapeutic target. *Intensive Care Med* **46(4):** 5 86-590.

Zhu LN, Mei X, Zhang, ZG, Xie YP, Lang, F (2019) Curcumin intervention for cognitive function in different types of people: a systematic review and meta-analysis. *Phytother* Res **33:** 524–533.

Immunity Boosting Functional Foods to Combat COVID-19, Pages: 47–52
Edited by: Apurba Giri
Copyright © 2021, Narendra Publishing House, Delhi, India

C H A P T E R - 4

USE OF ASHWAGANDHA TO BOOST IMMUNITY TO COMBAT COVID-19

Khokan Chandra Gayen[1], Prabir Jana[2] and Apurba Giri[3]*

[1]*Ex-Student, Department of Nutrition,*
Mugberia Gangadhar Mahavidyalya, PO-Bhupatinagar,
Dist. - Purba Medinipur- 721425, West Bengal, India
E-mail: chandragayen113@gmail.com
[2]*State Aided College Teacher,*
Department of Nutrition,
Mugberia Gangadhar Mahavidyalya, PO-Bhupatinagar,
Dist. - Purba Medinipur- 721425, West Bengal, India
E-mail: janaprabir113@gmail.com
[3]*Assistant Professor & Head, Department of Nutrition, Coordinator,*
Dept. of Food Processing, Mugberia Gangadhar Mahavidyalaya, P.O-Bhupatinagar;
Dist. - Purba Medinipur-721425, West Bengal, India
E-mail: apurbandri@gmail.com
*Corresponding author

ABSTRACT

The use of Ashwagandha plant extracts may be helpful due to its defensive antibody against virus like corona virus. In this time world is suffering from COVID-19. It has become crucial to keep ourself safe and healthy. Ashwagandha may be recommended for use as positive immunomodulator and it can also be used to destroy the COVID-19 virus. Despite, the ambiguity, it can be said that Ashwagandha is safe enough to use as an herbal remedy for COVID-19 prevention. Now the Ashwagandha food products (Ashwagandha tea, coffee, moonmilk, honey etc) may control the COVID-19 disease.

Keywords: Ashwagandha plant, COVID-19 virus, Immunomodulator.

INTRODUCTION

In this time world is under COVID-19. It has become crucial to be in safe and healthy. Even though we have come to know a lot about this new strain of the virus in this year, we are far away from getting an effective cure from the highly contagious disease, apart from practicing social distancing, proper hand hygiene and wearing musk. Ashwagandha is a plethora of health benefits, such as lowering stress and anxiety, reducing inflammation etc. In Ayurveda, Ashwagandha is mostly used herbs. Now, research suggests that the ayurvedic herb can be an effective as therapeutic and preventive drug against COVID -19. The root of the Ashwagandha plant has therapeutic benefit and has an effect on the nervous system. This is very helpful in the treatment of depression, anxiety, fatigue, stress induced insomnia and nervous exhaustion. Parts of this tree as root and leaves are used as medicine and it also a good source of minerals and dietary fiber. Several biochemical compounds present in roots are tyrosine, sominine, potassium, lactones, glucosides, withanolids, tannins, somniferine, iron, acyl sterile glucosides. Ashwagandha have various health benefit and it also used to treatment of many disese like diabetes, relieves stress, control air fall, boosts immunity, reduce ocular disease, control blood cholesterol level, increase blood production, have anti-microbial and anti-inflammatory properties. These herbs contain several micro and macro nutrients like glycowithanolides, iron tannins, alkaloids, fatty acids, glucose, potassium nitrate and other substances.

The Ashwagandha plant is a small sharp with yellow flowers that is native to India and North Africa. Extracts or powder from the plant roots or leaves is used to treat of variety of condition like it reduces the blood sugar level, reduces the stress hormone etc. The extracts of the powder root of the Ashwagandha is made to stimulate the immunological activity. Ashwagandha extracts inhabits hypersensitive response in rat. The immune-stimulants are T or the complement system rise in phagocytosis by the macrophages and granulocyte plays the central role in the immune-stimulation. Ashwagandha is a medicinal plant which is popular as home remedy for the several disease and human requirements. It is in use for a very long time for all age group and both sex and even during pregnancy without any side effects. The effect of this medicinal plant on various level nonspecific immune mechanism and cellular response has not been extensively studied. Activation of macrophage is perhaps important for the stimulating agent to remind in contact with the responsive cell (Honda, 2019).

Our daily requirements of energy and nutrients come from food. For the prevention and treatment of various diseases, foods are fortified with natural herbs and their bioactive (Yance, 2013). Due to health beneficial effect of Ashwagandha, it is used for the fortification of food and it is available in market as powder form. Hence, there is need to develop more Ashwagandha added fortified food to its health beneficial effect. Due to its bitter taste it can't consumed in raw form.

Botanical Description

➢ **The profile of Plant**

Family	Solanaceae
Name of Ayurvedic	Ashvagangha
Name of Unain	Asgand, AsgandNagori
Name of Hindi	Asgandh
Name of English	Winter Cherry
Name of Trade	Ashwagandha
Used of Parts	Root, Leaf and Seed

➢ **Morphological Characteristics** (Masanovic, 2019)

- It is solid haired, steep grayish-tomentose herb or underbush be on the increases to a height of 1.5 meter tall.
- Its all parts are overwhelmed with whitish, stellate trichomes.
- Branching is extensive; leaves are simple, interchange or sub-opposite, ovate entire, 10cm tall.
- The roots are stout, tall bulbaceous, fleshy, whitish- brown.

➢ **Immunomodulation:** Improvement of clinical and empirical immunology sharply expressed that multiple infectious, viral disease and disorder appeared because in stressful condition of environment attached with grip of immune system. It's clear evident that sure character of stress evoke physically changes that impact of malignance and infection to susceptibility. To modify of power the immune repercussion in humans and animals developed from hope to delegate greater defense against infectious agents and viral agents like a corona virus through a more full understanding of the function of the immune system, and of ways in which specific and non-specific immune mechanisms promoted. Naturally happen or artificial compounds able of changing those mechanisms offered further chance for modifying immune responses (Whitaker, 2017).

➢ **Mechanism of immune-stimulation:** Immunological defence is a complex interplay between specific and non-specific, cellular and humoral immune responses, stimulus and compression of immune competent cells, and the influence of endocrine and other mechanisms upon the immune system. Basic goals of Immuno stimulant are T or B lymphocytes or the complement system, raise in phagocytosis by macrophages and granulocytes plays central role in immuno-stimulation (Owen, 2011). Activation of macrophages is perhaps important for the stimulating agent to remain in contact with the responsive cell. On 2nd most significant role is the stimulation of T lymphocytes, which can be fulfilled either directly or indirectly, via macrophage (Gordon and Martinez, 2010).

➢ **Immunostimulant:** The immuno-stimulation includes a prophylactic or therapeutic opinion which aims at the stimulation of our non-specific immune system. This signifies primarily the non-antigen dependant stimulation of the behaviour and ability of work of glanulocytes, macrophages, complement and natural killer (NK) cells (Pavic, 2010).

Use of Ashwagandha

As a food (Alamgir, 2018)

➢ **Ashwagandha Tea**
-   To fight depression, anxiety, boost fertility and brain functioning.
-   It help to induce apoptosis, which is programmed death of cancer cells. It is used as an anticancer drug.

➢ **Ashwagandha coffee:** It is used to treatment the people for their day to day woes such as stress, anxiety, lack of sleep. It helps to block the stress pathway in the brain.

➢ **Ashwagandha chawanprash:** It is known as antibacterial agent. It increases the natural killer cell in the human body which are immuno cell that fight against infection.

➢ **Ashwagandha moon milk:** It is anti-inflammatory, antioxidant product. It decreases the C Reactive Protein in blood that increases the inflammation. It also decreases the cortisol hormone so free radicals production is less than normal production in human body.

➢ **Ashwagandha Honey:** It is an immunobooster. It also increases the natural killer cell in the blood. It also helps to fight against infection.

As a Medicine

➢ **Ashwagandha 60**
-   Adoptogen
-   Promotes the healthy stress response
➢ **Ashwagandha 120**
-   Destroy the free radicals
-   Promotes the good health

➤ **PET Ashwagandha 120**
- Provide the brain support
- Support the thyroid gland

➤ **Organic Ashwagandha:** Provide stress relief by supporting adrenals and balance the cortisol.

➤ **Ashwagandha Capsules**
- Build immunity
- Preventing cold, flu, bronchitis.
- Used anti-inflammatory agent.

CONCLUSION

The use of Ashwagandha plant extracts in particular dose time of the predetermined vaccination regimen may be helpful in presence higher defensive antibody against virus like a COVID-19 virus. Because Ashwagandha helps us to grow the cell's mediate immune response activity in our body. Ashwagandha may be recommended for use as positive immunomodulator and it can also be used to destroy the COVID-19 virus. It is more effective for therapeutic applications because it's high efficacy, low cost and low toxicity.

Ashwagandha food products are strong aphrodisiac with oxidative stress relieving and healing property which acts as an antioxidant in the cells boosting our immunity. Because of this rejuvenating property, it is widely used in different virus disease treatment. Now the same Ashwagandha health benefits make it one of the most promising immunity-boosting herb that can be used for COVID-19 prevention. The antioxidant properties have a certain antibacterial feature to it that prevents other associated virus infection.

Recent research highlights that Ashwagandha has certain chemical compounds called Withanone (Wi-N) that can block proteins which take part in viral replication, thus preventing the coronavirus from replicating and killing it.

Despite, the ambiguity, it is safe to say that Ashwagandha is enough to use as an herbal remedy for COVID-19 prevention. The Ashwagandha food products (Ashwagandha tea, coffee, moonmilk, honey etc.) may control the COVID-19 disease.

REFERENCES

Alamgir ANM (2018) Secondary Metabolites, **In:** Secondary Metabolic Products Consisting of C and H; C, H, and O; N, S, and P Elements; and O/N Heterocycles, **In:** Therapeutic Use of Medicinal Plants and their Extracts. Springer, Cham, Volume 2 (pp. 165-309).

Gordon S, Martinez FO (2010) Alternative activation of macrophages: mechanism and functions. *Immunity*, **32(5):** 593-604.

Honda M (2019) Reverse Heart Disease Naturally, **In:** Cures for high cholesterol, hypertension, arteriosclerosis, blood clots, aneurysms, myocardial infarcts and more. Hatherleigh Press.

Masanovic B (2019) Comparative Study of Morphological Characteristics and Body Composition between Different Team Players from Serbian Junior National League: Soccer, Handball, Basketball and Volleyball. *Int J Morphol* **37(2).**

Owen MAG (2011) The effect of dietary inclusion of category 3 animal by-product meals on rainbow trout (O. mykissWalbaum) mineralised tissues and immune function.

Pavic A (2010) The control of poultry Salmonella colonisation by vaccination and prophylactic treatment with anti-Salmonella antibodies.

Pradeu T (2011) The limits of the self: immunology and biological identity. Oxford University Press.

Saroj P, Verma M, Jha KK, Pal M (2012) An overview on immunomodulation. *J Adv Sci Res* **3(1):** 7-12.

Tizard IR (2017) Veterinary Immunology-E-Book. Elsevier Health Sciences.

Whitaker ED (2017) The Trouble with Human Nature, **In:** Health, Conflict, and Difference in Biocultural Perspective. Taylor & Francis.

Yance DR (2013) Adaptogens in medical herbalism, **In:** Elite herbs and natural compounds for mastering stress, aging, and chronic disease. Simon and Schuster.

Immunity Boosting Functional Foods to Combat COVID-19, Pages: 53–60
Edited by: Apurba Giri

CHAPTER - 5

BOOSTING IMMUNITY BY LIQUORICE (YASHTIMADHU) IN COVID-19 PANDEMIC SITUATION

Apurba Giri[1]*, Ashis Bera[2], Debabrata Giri[3] and Biswajit Das[4]

[1]*Assistant Professor & Head, E-mail: apurbandri@gmail.com*
[2]*Ex-Student, E-mail: ashisberabsc@gmail.com*
[3]*Ex-Student, E-mail: giridebabrata409@gmail.com*
[4]*Ex-Student, E-mail: dbiswajit649@gmail.com*
Dept. of Nutrition, Mugberia Gangadhar Mahavidyalaya, Bhupatinagar,
Purba Medinipur-721425, West Bengal, India
*Corresponding author

ABSTRACT

Corona virus disease 2019 (COVID-19) is caused due to corona virus that spreaded worldwide and became a pandemic. Currently several studies are going on to search appropriate drugs or vaccine to prevent these disease. To search the plant based medicines which have antiviral and Immunomodulatory properties that prevent the viral infected disease. Liquorice root is used worldwide as an herbal medicine. This root commonly known as sweet wood, Mulethi or Yashtimadhu. Various active components like glycyrrhizin, isoflavonoids, triterpenoids, sterol, amino acid etc that have antiviral and immunomodulatory properties. Liquorice has the ability to reduce the expression of proinflammatory cytokines, interleukin, TNFα, and stimulate the secretion of lymphocyte. SARS-Cov2 and SARS-CoV have the same receptor ACE2. Glycyrrhetinic acid helps to down regulate the expression of angiotensin-converting enzyme 2 (ACE2) in lungs and prevent the entry of virus. Liquorice polysaccharide helps to modulate our immune system by the activation of CD4 T cell. In this present study we reviewed about the Immunomodulatory effect of liquorice that helps in healthy living in pandemic situation.

Keywords: Liquorice, Immunomodulation, Glycyrrhizin, COVID-19, ACE2, CD4 T cell.

INTRODUCTION

World Health Organization declared that corona virus or COVID-19 create a pandemic situation all-over the world. This pandemic situation changes the daily lives of people and also changes the diet taking during COVID-19 pandemic. There are several foods like lemon, ghee, dates, various types of spicy, seeds and legumes, nuts etc that also improve our immunity and prevent various infected disease in this pandemic situation. To prevent the spread of the severe acute respiratory syndrome corona virus 2 (SARS-CoV-2) immediately needed effective medication but at present no treatment are available. Viral disease are spared vary quickly and are difficult to control this spreading due to their metabolic properties and quickly drug resistance power. Common medications are often inadequate and show a variety of side effects. In this situation we try to improve our immunity by taking proper diet. Natural remedies like herb are used to prevent various infected disease in both immune competent and immune compromised individuals (Perera and Efferth, 2012).

The World Health Organization (WHO) estimated that about an 80% population of developing countries relies on traditional medicines, mostly plant drugs, for their primary health care needs. Use of raw plant products that connect with Ayurvedic medicine are mostly used in Indian rural area because the availability of the raw plants in rural area is more (Anagha *et al.*, 2014). One of the most used herbal plants is liquorice or mulethi (in Hindi) or yashtimadhu (in Bengali) that have antiviral and antimicrobial properties. The enzyme present in liquorices root helps in boost our immunity naturally by producing lymphocyte and macrophages that protect our body from microbes, pollutants, allergens.

The scientific name of the liquorice is *Glycyrrhiza glabra* comes from the Fabaceae family. This plant is called 'sweet root' that's name comes from the scientific name 'Glycyrrhiza'. The term 'glykos' which means 'sweet' and the term 'rhiza' means 'root' and hence the name given to this plant is 'sweet root'. In Ayurveda 'Yashtimadhu' is the herb named as the word 'Yashti' means 'wood' and Madhu means 'honey' together making it 'honey-like wood'. In the presence of a chemical compound called glycyrrhizin the root is sweeter than sugar. Liquorice root have several secondary which is used to treatment various disease like cancer, tuberculosis, atherosclerosis, gastric ulcers, immunodeficiency hepatitis and this root also improve our immunity (Isbrucker and Burdock 2006; Kalani *et al.*, 2015). Several studies have shown that the chemical compound glycyrrhizic acid present in liquorice helps provoke T cells for production of IFN-γ. In a recent study it also showed that SARS-CoV2 and SARS- CoV have the same receptor site ACE2, glycyrrhizic acid can bind with this receptor and prevent the binding of this type of virus. Glycyrrhizic acid may have therapeutic effects on SARS-CoV-2 (Chen and Du, 2020).

Plant Description

Liquorice or licorice is the common name of Glycyrrhiza glabra, a flowering plant of fabaceae family. The outer surface of the liquorice root is yellowish-brown in color. After 2-3 years of plantation pale blue flowers are occurs.

Scientific classification (Anil and Joytsna, 2012)

Kingdom: Plantae

   Division: Angiospermae

      Class: Dicotyledonae

         Order: Rosales

            Family: Leguminosae

               Genus: Glycyrrhiza

               Species: glabra Linn

Vernacular names (Anagha *et al.,* 2012)

Sanskrit: Yashtimadhuka, Yashtika

English: Liquorice root

Bengali: Jashtimadhu

Hindi: Mulethi, Mulathi

Cultivated Area

Generally this plant is grown-up in dry, sunny climate and cultivated in warm temperature and subtropical region and mostly in Mediterranean region. Liquorice producing countries are India, Iran, Italy, Azerbaijan, China, Pakistan, Iraq, Uzbekistan, Afghanistan, Turkmenistan and Turkey (M & F Worldwide Corp, 2010). Cultivated in Jammu and Kashmir, Punjab and sub-Himalayan tracts in India (Hegde and Harini, 2014).

Chemical Constituents

Several bioactive compound present in this root are flavonoids, isoflavins, saponoids, sterols, various types of sugar, amino acid, essential oil and glycyrrhizin and that's have several health benefit and immunomodulatory effect on human. Liquorice contains more than 300 flavonoids and more than 20 tripinoids, among them mostly active compound are glycyrrhizin, liquiritigenin, 18β-glycyrrhetinic acid, liquiritigenin, glabridin which have antiviral and antimicrobial activities (Kokate *et al.*, 2004).

Immunomodulatory Effect

In COVID-19 pandemic situation there is no vaccine or medicinal treatment are available, so in this situation improve our immunity by various natural food or natural herbs to prevent viral infected disease. Liquorice can do wonders for our immunity naturally. Various phytochemicals present in the liquorice roots that stimulate the production of macrophages, lymphocytes that protect our body from virus and boost our immunity naturally. In this situation various therapies to affect the replication of virus (James *et al.*, 2020) one of these are immunotherapies that reduced the virus induced inflammation (Bonam *et al.*, 2020). Liquorice extract have the potential effect on to reduce the expression of proinflametory cytokines, interleukin 1(IL-1, IL-6) tumor necrosis factor (TNF-α) (Yu *et al.*, 2015). By the spike protein CoVs infect the host cell surface. SARS-CoV-2 have spike protein that is bind with the cellular receptor angiotensin-converting enzyme 2 (ACE2) and enter inside the cell (Zhang *et al.*, 2020). Many studies have shown that there is a strong association between SARS-Co-2 and human ACE2, the surface protein of many cell types. Glycyrrhizin present in liquorice have the potential effect, it binds with ACE2 active site and prevent binding of virus in active site of ACE2 (Chen and Du, 2020).

Liquorice has a polysaccharide acts on spleen and thymus that is the major secondary and primary lymphoid organs that involved in maturation of immune cell and it is also important in humoral and cellular immunity, it stimulate proliferation of T lymphocytes and enhance secretion of IL-7 (Ayeka *et al.*, 2016). One of the most active components of liquorice root is glycyrrhizin (GL) which metabolized in human gut and produced glycyrrhetinic acid (GA). GA inhibits enzyme called 11-beta-hydroxysteroid dehydrogenase, both type 1 and 2 (Cosmetic Ingredient Review Expert Panel, 2007). This inhibition allows cortisol to access mineralocorticoid receptor (MR) in aldosterone specific peripheral tissue present in lungs, kidney, nasal and endothelium cell, that's results the aldosterone level is increased by aldosterone like activation of MR via cortisol. High level of aldosterone lead to down regulate of ACE2 in kidney (Fukuda *et al.*, 2011), lungs, and nasal epithelium cell that's why the inhibition of main entry path of COVID-19 virus (Keidar *et al.*, 2005).

One of the most probable mechanisms for immunomodulation is the activation of immune cell as like CD4 and CD8 T cell. Liquorice polysaccharide has the ability to stimulate the proliferation of CD4 T cell and reduce the activity of CD8 T cell. CD4 T cell have anticancer properties (Marzo *et al.,* 2000; Assudani *et al.,* 2007) and have the ability to promote antitumor activity of CD8 T cell. Liquorice polysaccharide stimulate the activation of lymphocytes is a probable mechanism of immunomodulation (Gyobu *et al.,* 2004).

WAY OF CONSUMPTION

Liquorice Tea

Liquorice is most benefactions herbal product that consumed in various way, one of the most popular is liquorice tea. Liquorice contains a natural sweetener called glycyrrhizin that is sweeter than sucrose. Not only it has medicinal properties, it tastes also delicious. There is some limitation for consumption – one or two cup per day for medicinal purpose and should be used it under supervision of health professionals, because excessive consumption of liquorice have various side effects. For the preparation of liquorice tea ingredients - 1 inch liquorice root, 2 cups water, few sliced lime pieces are required. At first water are boiled then liquorice root is added and allowed boiling for a few minutes, then strained into a cup and adding lemon slices.

Liquorice Candy

Liquorice extract is produced from the roots of liquorice plant *Glycyrrhiza glabra* and it is used as a confection usually flavour and black colour. Liquorice is widly used in various sweet products. Black liquorice confectionary is available in market and its main ingredient is liquorice extract, sugar and a binding agent like starch, geletin, gum Arabic. Anise oil is used in liquorice candy for improvement of flavour (US Food & Drug Administration, 2011). For the preparation of this product at first all ingredients are boiled with water at 135°C. Then liquid is poured into molds. A shiny surface of sweet is prepared after drying of liquid portion. Red liquorice is also produced by adding strawberry, raspberry, and cherry or cinnamon that also improves flavour of the product.

Preparation of Liquorice Powder at Home

For preparation of various food products, liquorice powder is used and the powder is stored several days in cool places at air tight container. For this preparation at first the root is washed with water to remove the soil and other impurities then fresh root of liquorice is cut into pieces. It is dried under direct sunlight for some weeks until there is no moisture left. The dried roots are ground in a grinder and produce a fine powder. It is stored in an air tight containers in cool places for future use

CONCLUSION

Liquorice is widely used as a traditional herbal medicine. Many active compound present in liquorice that have potential role in treatment of various disease and have antimicrobial properties that protect our body from virus infected disease. In this chapter we have discussed the immunomodulatory effect of liquorice. It have capability to reduce the expression of ACE2 in lungs and prevent the entry of virus in body through respiratory tract, liquorice also stimulate the lymphocyte production and modulate the immune system. In COVID-19 pandemic situation improve our immune function is the only way to prevent the attack of virus until vaccine are available in market. Liquorice has antimicrobial and immunomodulatory properties but there is more scientific studies are required to explore these properties to combat COVID-19.

REFERENCES

Anagha K, Manasi D, Priya L, Meera M (2012) comprehensive review on historical aspect of yashtimadhu-glycyrrhiza glabra L. *Global J Res Med Plants Indigen Med* **1(12):687.**

Anagha K, Manasi D, Priya L, Meera M (2014) Antimicrobial activity of Yashtimadhu (Glycyrrhiza glabra L.)-A Review. *Int J Curr Microbiol App Sci* **3(1):** 329-336.

Anil K, Jyotsna D (2012) Review on *Glycyrrhiza glabra* (Liquorice). *J Pharm Sci Innov* **1(2):**1-4.

Assudani DP, Horton RB, Mathieu MG, McArdle SE, Rees RC (2007) The role of CD4+ T cell help in cancer immunity and the formulation of novel cancer vaccines. *Cancer Immunol Immunother* **56(1):**70–80.

Ayeka PA, Bian Y, Mwitari PG, Chu X, Zhang Y, Uzayisenga R, Otachi EO (2016) Immunomodulatory and anticancer potential of Gan cao (*Glycyrrhiza uralensis* Fisch.) polysaccharides by CT-26 colon carcinoma cell growth inhibition and cytokine IL-7 upregulation in vitro. *BMC Complement Altern Med* **16(1):** 206.

Black Licorice: Trick or Treat? From US Food & Drug Administration, Consumer Updates, 25 Oct 2011.

Bonam SR, Kaveri SV, Sakuntabhai A, Gilardin L, Bayry J (2020) Adjunct immunotherapies for the management of severely ill COVID-19 patients. *Cell Rep Med*, 100016.

Chen H, Du Q (2020) Potential natural compounds for preventing SARS-CoV-2 (2019-nCoV) infection. *Preprints*: 202001.0358.v32020010358.

Cosmetic Ingredient Review Expert Panel (2007) Final report on the safety assessment of Glycyrrhetinic Acid, Potassium Glycyrrhetinate, Disodium Succinoyl Glycyrrhetinate, Glyceryl Glycyrrhetinate, Glycyrrhetinyl Stearate, Stearyl Glycyrrhetinate, Glycyrrhizic Acid, Ammonium Glycyrrhizate, Dipotassium Glycyrrhizate, Disodium Glycyrrhizate, Trisodium Glycyrrhizate, Methyl Glycyrrhizate, and Potassium Glycyrrhizinate *Int J Toxicol 26*:79.

Fukuda S, Horimai C, Harada K, Wakamatsu T, Fukasawa H, Muto S, ... Hayashi M (2011) Aldosterone-induced kidney injury is mediated by NFκB activation. *Clin Exp Nephrol 15(1)*: 41-49.

Gyobu H, Tsuji T, Suzuki Y, Ohkuri T, Chamoto K, Kuroki M, Miyoshi H, Kawarada Y, Katoh H, Takeshima T (2004) Generation and targeting of human tumor-specific Tc1 and Th1 cells transduced with a lentivirus containing a chimeric immunoglobulin T-cell receptor. Cancer Res. *64(4)*: 1490–5.

Hegde DPL, Harini DA (2014) A Textbook of Dravyaguna Vijnana.

Isbrucker RA, Burdock GA. (2006) Risk and safety assessment on the consumption of Licorice root (Glycyrrhiza sp.), its extract and powder as a food ingredient, with emphasis on the pharmacology and toxicology of glycyrrhizin. *Regul Toxicol Pharmacol 46(3)*: 167-192.

James M, Marguerite L, Tomasz Z, James B (2020) Pharmacologic treatments for coronavirus disease 2019 (COVID 19). *JAMA 323(18)*: 1824-1836.

Kalani K, Chaturvedi V, Alam S, Khan F, Kumar Srivastava S (2015) Anti-tubercular agents from Glycyrrhiza glabra. *Curr Top Med Chem 15(11)*: 1043-1049.

Keidar S, Gamliel-Lazarovich A, Kaplan M, Pavlotzky E, Hamoud S, Hayek T et al. (2005) Mineralocorticoid receptor blocker increases angiotensin-converting enzyme 2 activity in congestive heart failure patients. *Circ Res 97*: 946–53.

Kokate CK, Purohit AP, Gokhale SB (2004) The Text book of Pharmacognosy, Nirali Prakashan, 28th edition, Pune, Maharashtra, India, pp 212–215.

M & F Worldwide Corp., Annual Report on Form 10-K for the Year Ended December 31, 2010.

Marzo AL, Kinnear BF, Lake RA, Frelinger JJ, Collins EJ, Robinson BW, Scott B (2000) Tumor-specific CD4+ T cells have a major "post-licensing" role in CTL mediated anti-tumor immunity. *J Immunol 165(11)*: 6047–55.

Perera C, EfferthT (2012) Antiviral medicinal herbs and phytochemicals. *J Pharmacogn 3*(**1**): 45-48.

Yu JY, Ha JY, Kim KM, Jung YS, Jung JC, Oh S (2015) Anti-inflammatory activities of licorice extract and its active compounds, glycyrrhizic acid, liquiritin and liquiritigenin, in BV2 cells and mice liver. *Molecules 20*(**7**): 13041-13054.

Zhang H, Penninger JM, Li Y, Zhong N, Slutsky AS (2020) Angiotensin-converting enzyme 2 (ACE2) as a SARS-CoV-2 receptor: molecular mechanisms and potential therapeutic target. *Inten care Med* **46**(**4**): 586-590.

Immunity Boosting Functional Foods to Combat COVID-19, Pages: 61–74
Edited by: Apurba Giri
Copyright © 2021, Narendra Publishing House, Delhi, India

CHAPTER - 6

ROLE OF INDIAN HERBS IN BOOSTING IMMUNITY

Preeti Bora

Academic Associate, Department of Home Science, School of Health Sciences
Uttarakhand Open University, Haldwani-263139, Uttarakhand, India
E-mail: borapreeti@gmail.com

ABSTRACT

The world today is badly affected with the deadly Corona virus. Boosting the body's immunity has gained a sudden and intense attention globally as people with better immune are reported to be less affected. Apart from the immunity boosting preparations that people consume, a major role has been played by food in building a better immune mechanism of the body. Protection from different viral and bacterial infections is a vital role of strong immunity. Presently many herbs are being used in different ailments and this trend is increasing rapidly. Many herbs that we use in our day-to-day lives are helpful in boosting the immunity thus helpful in fighting infections. The pungent-smelling herb Garlic, has antibiotic, anti-inflammatory and antimicrobialproperties and is found to have some compounds that boost the disease-fighting response of some particular white blood cells when they encounter viruses. The extracts or powder of leaves and roots of *Ashwagandha* can reduce blood sugar and cortisol levels, symptoms of depression and helps in increasing strength and muscle mass. *Tulsi* is an immunity boosting herb, which helps in relieving many lung-related diseases and is also beneficial in cramping, gastric disorders, reducing sugar, controlling blood pressure and skin-related problems. *Amla* is full of antioxidants primarily Vitamin C that is helpful in detoxifying the entire organ system for better health and immunity. *Neem* is another antimicrobial herb whose every part is therapeutic in nature. With detoxification effect on the body it also has the capability to fight fungus, viruses and bacteria. The active compound of turmeric; curcumin found to have anti-inflammatory and antioxidant properties. Ginger has antibacterial properties. Gingerol is a phenolic anti-inflammatory compound found in ginger that helps in relaxing blood vessels and functions as natural blood thinner. Many other herbs like Cinnamon, *Giloy*, Black pepper, Cloves have important roles in boosting immunity. This paper undertakes a review of available contemporary and basic literature on the role of different herbs in increasing human immunity which can be helpful to stay healthy during this pandemic.

Keywords: COVID-19, Coronavirus, Immunity, Indian herbs, Immunomodulators, Herbal medicine.

INTRODUCTION

Corona viruses are big family of viruses which may cause ill effect on health of humans. Several respiratory infections causing corona viruses are identified. These may cause many ailments in humans which could be common cold to more severe like Severe Acute Respiratory Syndrome (SARS). The most recently discovered corona virus is COVID-19. Its outbreak first reported in December 2019 in Wuhan, China (Ministry of Health and Family Welfare, GOI, 2020). Mild to moderate sickness is reported commonly in people infected with COVID-19 virus and they don't require any special treatment for its cure.

World Health Organization and respective national guidelines related to prevention and slowing down spread of COVID has been issued to let people all over the world know about coronavirus, the disease it causes and how it spreads (World Health Organization, 2020).

Corona viruses (CoV) were mainly known as causative agents of mild respiratory and gastrointestinal disease until the SARS outbreak in 2002, where this family of virus displayed its potential for wide spread and significant pathogenicity in humans. The recent addition to human pathogenic coronaviruses (hCoVs) is SARS-CoV2 which is the cause of COVID-19 that has affected people worldwide. As the immunity against this virus does not exist in humans so its unrestricted proliferation could happen in primarily infected tissues. Following the death of the cells, the virus particles and intracellular components releases in extracellular spaces that result in the generation of immune complexes, immune cell recruitment and allied damage (Felsenstein *et al.*, 2020).

Enhancing the body's natural defense system (immunity) plays an important role in maintaining optimum health. As of now there is no apposite medicine/vaccine for COVID-19, taking appropriate preventive measures is advisable which could enhance our immunity as prevention is better than cure (Ministry of AYUSH, GOI, 2020). Many herbs that we use in our day-to-day lives are helpful in boosting the immunity thus helpful in fighting infections. The rationale of this review paper is to provide a comprehensive summary of the current scientific literature on the effect of different herbs in increasing human immunity which can be helpful to stay healthy during the current pandemic; COVID-19.

The Immune System

Boosting the body's immunity has gained a sudden and intense attention globally as people with better immune are reported to be less affected with this virus. Strong immunity plays a crucial role in protecting from different viral and bacterial infections. The key players in the immune system are the white blood cells that can travel all over the body through blood cells to watch for microbes that invades the body. This cycle is continued all over by watching over foreign antigens and then progressively floats again in lymphatic system. The immune cells gather in lymph nodes and compartments of spleen to work against the antigens (Chowdhury et al., 2020).

The immune system of body comprises of many biological units like cells, tissues and organs. The immune system protects the body form many external threats like microorganisms (bacteria, viruses, and parasites), their deadly products like exotoxins and endotoxins. This immune mechanism also protects the body from external air or food-borne allergens. Likewise there are many internal threats too like the microorganisms found in various body systems (skin, gut, respiratory and urogenital system). Innate and adaptive immunity are two major functional components of the immune system. Whenever the body is exposed to some antigen the innate immunity protects the body from its harmful effects. Innate immunity cannot be adapted (Kussmann, 2010). The body's immunity is a complex system. It can act both naturally and acquired, although most of the time it is in collaboration. One of the important factors affecting the immune system of body is nutrition. Malnutrition curbs the immune system. There are various nutrients in our food that play important role in boosting the immunity and maintaining a healthy immune system. Foods rich in protein, vitamins like C and E and various minerals like zinc, selenium, magnesium helps in boosting the body's immunity against various pathogens (Karacabey and Ozdemir, 2012).

Nutrition and Immunity

Malnutrition is the most common reason for immunodeficiency globally and a healthy immune response needs a healthy diet with balanced nutrition. Many studies have backed the fact that nutritional deficiencies can alter one's immune competency and thus can increase risk of infections.

Of all the macronutrients, carbohydrate is required for stimulation/functioning of immune system. Carbohydrate is needed for constant supply of energy to cells and tissues. Carbohydrate can minimize the collection of many cells for cell death thus making it an essential component in the immunity system. Fats are dense energy source. Fatty acids act as potent modulators of the body's immune response. Linoleic acid decreases allergic sensitization. Omega-3 fatty acids lower plasma aggregation, blood pressure and inflammatory response. They can also control immune responses pertaining to cells.

The chemical structure of protein contains carbon, hydrogen, nitrogen and oxygen. For many immune mechanisms, active protein compounds production or cell replication is a relying factor. Functions of immune system decrease in protein deficiency. Deficiency of essential amino acids can also cause oppression on immune system. An important role is played by protein metabolism in immune responses. It plays a key role in development of body's immunity against many infections (Karacabey and Ozdemir, 2012).

Among B group, many vitamins like riboflavin, pyridoxine, cyanocobalamin and folate are helpful on immune system. Pyridoxine is the most desired vitamin for immune system. Vitamin B12 and folic acid are strongly associated to the immune mechanism. They have important role in protein, DNA and RNA synthesis. In conditions where there is deficiency of vitamin pyridoxine, there is less production of lymphocytes and immunity cells that have a negative impact on the response of body's immune response against infections (Greiner, 2011).

Vitamin C or ascorbic acid act against infections from bacteria and the ill effects of their toxins. Studies have found that there is an increase in white blood cell production with supplementation of ascorbic acid. Dietary iron absorption increases with the supplementation of vitamin C. It is also known as an anticancer factor because of its antioxidative properties. (Karacabey and Ozdemir, 2012).

Vitamin A has anti inflammatory effect. It plays a key role in formation of epithelial tissues and in visual functions. It also provides strength to the immune system of body (Reifen, 2002).

Vitamin D has also considerable effect on the body's immune mechanism. It has been demonstrated that innate and adaptive immune systems can be modulated by vitamin D. Both immune systems are adjusted by vitamin D, which suppresses the adaptive immune system but potent the innate immune processes. Vitamin D has reinforcing and inhibitory effects for both immune mechanisms, respectively. It has anti-inflammatory properties and modulates immunity in different ways and is effective in physiology and autoimmunity (Nilashi et al., 2020).

The antioxidant function of vitamin E makes it primarily effective against infections. Vitamin E inhibits the production of platelets and immune modulators and in this way it enhances the immune response to infections and external agents. Both selenium and zinc are required for stimulation of sound immune response. For a healthy immune system development and its prolongation, copper plays a key role. Immune system is affected by both the deficiency and abundance of iron. Bacteria and virus both need iron for their proliferation. So during acute infections, iron should be avoided. During the conditions when iron is deficient in the body, less number of white blood cells transported towards the infectious area. Therefore the microorganisms entering in the cells could not be damaged (Chandra, 2003).

Indian Herbs as Immunity Boosters

There is a rapid growth in the use of herbs for the treatment of different ailments. Many herbs that we use in our day-to-day lives are helpful in boosting the immunity thus helpful in fighting infections. At a time when the world is coping with the deadly corona virus, extra precautions are necessary to keep ourselves protected from infections. The COVID-19 pandemic has made people observant about the role of immunity in fighting infections and thus stressed upon the role and use of kitchen herbs as immunity boosters. Ministry of AYUSH, Government of India has also suggested the use of *Dalchini* (Cinnamon), *Tulsi* (Basil), *Kali mirch* (Black pepper), *Haldi* (turmeric) and *Shunthi* (Dry Ginger) as ayurvedic immunity promoting measures.

Many Indian herbs are used as a treatment option primarily in many ailments. Herb refers to any part of the plant like fruit, seed, stem, bark, flower, leaf, stigma or a root, as well as a non-woody plant. WHO (World Health Organization) estimated that 80 percent of people worldwide rely on herbal medicines for some aspect of their primary health care needs. According to WHO, around 21,000 plant species can be used as medicinal plants for treating/preventing numerous ailments (National Health Portal, GOI). The role of few Indian herbs in modulating and boosting immune system of our body will be discussed in this review.

Garlic *(Allium sativum)*

Garlic is a widely consumed spice in the world. Garlic and its derivatives have many health benefits. It plays a role in maintaining the immune system homeostasis. It contains diverse bioactive compounds, such as allicin, diallyl sulfide, alliin, diallyl disulfide, diallyltrisulfide, ajoene, and S-allyl-cysteine (Shang *et al.*, 2019). These compounds from garlic when extracted and isolated, display many beneficial effects against infections from bacteria. Garlic compounds perform antiparasitic, antiapoptotic, anticancerigenic and immunomodulatory effects on different cells. Components present in garlic stimulate macrophages, natural killer cells, dendritic cells, lymphocytes and eosinophils. Garlic components modulate the secretion of cytokine and immunoglobulin production. They also stimulate phagocytosis and activate macrophages. This way they boost the immunity (Arreola *et al.*, 2015). Garlic is a rich natural source of bioactive sulfur-containing compounds and has promising applications in functional foods development or nutraceuticals for the management and prevention of certain diseases and help in boosting the immune system (Salman *et al.*, 1999).

Ashwagandha (*Withania somnifera*)

Ashwagandha is a much valued herb of Indian Ayurveda as Rasayana (tonic). It is used a tonic for nervous system related problems. In Ayurveda, it is one of the main herbal ingredients in tonics for elderly. It has general animating and regenerative qualities. *Ashwagandha* is used in treating nervous exhaustion, insomnia, memory related conditions, tiredness, potency issues, skin related problems and coughing. It improves memory capacity and learning ability (Verma and Kumar, 2011). *Ashwagandha* have anti-inflammatory, anti-oxidative, antimicrobial, anti-anxiety, immunomodulation, hypoglycaemic, anticancer, hypolipidemic properties. *Ashwagandha* is proved to be very effective in parkinson's and alzheimer's diseases (Jana and Madhu Charan, 2018).

Davis and Kuttan (2000) studied the immunomodulatory activity of *Withania somnifera* and found that it was found to enhance total WBC count and bone marrow cells significantly indicating that the extract could stimulate the haemopoetic system. Its extracts increase the levels of circulating antibody and antibody forming cells.

Tulsi (*Ocimum sanctum*)

Tulsi is believed to purify expectorants and called the "wonder herb". The roots, leaves and seeds of *Tulsi* possess several medicinal properties. Ayurvedictexts categorize *Tulsi* as stimulant, aromatic and antipyretic. It has a variety of pharmacological functions like anti protozoal, anti malarial, antipyretic, anti inflammatory, anti allergic, chemopreventive, immunomodulatory, anti stressand anticoagulant activities (Sai Krishna *et al.*, 2014).

Tulsi has antibacterial, antiviral and antifungal properties that include activity against many pathogens responsible for human infections. It boosts defenses against infective threats by enhancing immune responses in animals and healthy humans. *Tulsi* may aid in treating various human bacterial infections including UTIs (urinary tract infections), skin and wound infections, typhoid fever, cholera, tuberculosis, acne, herpes simplex, various pneumonias and fungal infections. Its unique combination of many properties *i.e.* antibacterial, analgesic, antioxidant and anti-inflammatory also makes it useful in wound healing (Cohen, 2014).

Active ingredients present in *Tulsi* have anti-inflammatory properties. It also plays a role in modulation of cellular and humeral immunity both. Taking *Tulsi* leaves on empty stomach found to increase immunity. It is used for immune-based therapies specially for treating various diseases. The alcoholic leaf extract of *Tulsi* shows immunomodulatory effect such as modulation of cytokine secretion, immunoglobulin secretion, histamine release, class switching, cellular co-receptor expression, phagocytosis and lymphocyte expression (Upadhyay, 2017).

Amla (*Emblica officinalis*)

Amla or Indian Gooseberry is widely used in the Ayurveda and is believed to increase body immune against diseases. Raw fruits of *Amla* have laxative effect; while the dried fruits are useful in inflammation, haemorrhage, cough, diarrhoea and dysentery, and in combination with iron, used for anaemia, jaundice and dyspepsia. The flowers have cooling, refrigerant and laxative effect; while theroot and bark are astringent. Its seeds are used for asthma, bronchitis and biliousness. *Amla* fruit contains ellagic and gallic acid, quercetin, emblicanin, flavonoids, kaempferol, glycosides and proanthocyanidins. Vitamin C (ascorbic acid), tannins and flavonoids present in *Amla* have very powerful antioxidant, immunomodulatory and anticancer activities. Quercetin present in *Amla* has hepatoprotective effect (Madhuri, 2011).

One reason for *Amla*'s standing as a general energy-boosting and disease-preventing tonic may be its effect on the body's immunity mechanism. Various studies have shown significant increase in white blood cell count and other measures of strengthened immunity in rodents given *Amla* (Grover *et al.*, 2015). Chyavnaprash which constitutes 70% 0f the *Amla* formulations is believed to be an immune enhancer and a health tonic for both children and elders (Srivasuki, 2012).

Neem (*Azadirachta indica*)

Neem is an evergreen tropical tree well known for its medicinal significance. Advantageous effects of different parts of *Neem* are attributed to its biologically active principle 'Azadirachtin'. The leaves of *Neem* have flavonoids, isoprenoids, polyphenols, sulphurous and polysaccharides that play a role in scavenging the free radical and subsequently apprehending disease pathogenesis (Yadav *et al.*,

2016). Leaf, blossom and stem bark extricates of *Neem* have strong antioxidant potential. Flavanoids present in *Neem* have a pivotal role in control of malignant growth advancement (Giri *et al.*, 2019). Immuno stimulating properties of *Neem* are its most critical advantage. It helps the "Killer T" cells which can destroy organisms, infections and malignancy cells by introducing poisonous synthetic compounds into the intruders thus support both the lymphocytic and cell-intervened frameworks (Mukherjee *et al.*, 2014).

Turmeric *(Curcuma longa)*

Due to its bright and lustrous yellow color, turmeric is also known as "Indian Saffron". It is an herb commonly used as a spice in Indian cuisine. Turmeric contains volatile and non-volatile oils in varied proportions depending on its origin and conditions of growth. It also consists of proteins, fats, minerals, carbohydrates, moisture and curcuminoids. Three molecules together of curcuminoids are called as curcumin. It is the most significant component found in turmeric having a percentage of 60 to 70 percent. The role of curcumin in the prevention and cure of various diseases like cardiovascular, inflammatory, cancer, neurological, skin related and metabolic are supported by various studies (Catanzaro *et al.*, 2018). Curcumin found in turmeric also have immunomodulatory ability which originates from its action in close association with different immunomodulators including both cellular (macrophages,dendritic cells and B &T lymphocytes) and molecular components (cytokines and transcription factors) involved in inflammation (Momtazi-Borojeni *et al.*, 2018). It is a potent immunomodulatory agent that can modulate the activation of T cells, B cells, macrophages, neutrophils, natural killer cells, and dendritic cells. Curcumin can also down regulate the expression of various proinflammatory cytokines and chemokines. It can also enhance antibody responses even at low doses (Jagetia and Aggarwal, 2007).

Curcumin is also known for its radical scavenging and antioxidant properties. It is mainly involved in scavenging of free radicals in peroxidation processes. Therefore, possessing a great potency to inhibit peroxidation of lipid and protect cell membrane from oxidative damage by positioning itself within the cell membrane. It is also considered as a potential antioxidant against hydrogen peroxide and superoxide radical generation (Boroumand *et al.*, 2018).

Ginger *(Zingiber officinale)*

Ginger is an herb indigenous to South-East Asia which is used as a spice and condiment. In addition to this the rhizome of ginger has medicinal properties too which make its use suitable in various traditional herbal medicines. The health-promoting perspective of ginger is credited to its rich phytochemistry (Mashhad *et al.*, 2013).

A variety of degenerative disorders like arthritis and rheumatism, cardiovascular ailments like atherosclerosis and hypertension and problems related to digestive health like indigestion, constipation and ulcer can be treated with the use of ginger. In addition it is also helpful in vomiting, diabetes mellitus, and cancer treatments. It has anti-inflammatory and anti-oxidative properties that make it useful in treatment of ailments.

Ginger can also be used in treating infections pertaining to its antimicrobial potential. The bioactive molecules of ginger like gingerols have antioxidant activity in various sections (Zheng and Wang, 2001). Ginger can help in the cure of inflammatory chronic diseases such as fatty liver, asthma, cancer and arthritis through anti-inflammatory, antioxidative and immunoregulatory mechanisms (Aryaeian and Tavakkoli, 2015).

Cinnamon (*Cinnamomum verum*)

Majorly used as spice and for adding flavor to food, cinnamon is an important compound in Ayurveda. The essential oil of the cinnamon bark constitutes more than 80% of cinnamaldehyde and the aqueous extract of the cinnamon spice has been attributed with antioxidant properties.

The anti-bacterial, anti-inflammatory, hypoglycemic, anti-mutagenic and anti-tumorigenic activity of cinnamon is attributed to a bioactive compound Cinnamaldehyde (CA) found in it. The immunomodulatory properties of cinnamon have been demonstrated by various in vitro and in vivo studies (Gruenwald *et al.*, 2010).

Giloy (*Tinospora cordifolia*)

T. cordifolia, commonly known as Guduchi or *Giloy*, is used as a medicine in the Ayurvedic and Unani systems of the medicine for centuries. *Giloy* extract contains many constituents such as alkaloids, steroids, glycosides, and polysaccharides. *Giloy* possess antioxidant, antidiabetic, antihepatotoxic, immunomodulatory properties (Panchabhai *et al.*, 2008). It is a well known immune-modulator herb used in the correction of auto immunity (Rawat and Roushan, 2018).

Giloy is used to improve or boost immunity. *Giloy* has found to have antioxidative properties that keep the body cells healthy and disease free by fighting free radicals circulating in the body. *Giloy* helps to remove toxins and purifies blood, fights against bacteria. The active compounds found in plant extract in the form of alkaloids, lactones, glycosides and steroids have immune modulatory role in the body (Saxena and Rawat, 2019).

Black pepper (*Piper nigrum*)

Vine and extracts of black pepper are used for their medicinal properties in many cultures. The chemical piperine is a major bioactive component present in black pepper that has numerous reported physiological and drug-like actions (Singletary, 2010).

Black pepper is an important healthy food owing to its antioxidant, antimicrobial potential and gastro-protective modules. Piperine in black pepper is an active ingredient that holds rich phytochemistry including volatile oil, oleoresins, and alkaloids. The free-radical scavenging activity of black pepper and its active ingredients might be helpful in chemoprevention and controlling progression of tumor growth. Additionally, the key alkaloid components i.e. piperine assists in cognitive brain functioning, boost nutrient's absorption and improve gastrointestinal functionality. In Indian folklore medicine, it is mainly used as an immune enhancer and to treat against diarrhea, asthma, chronic indigestion, gastric ailments (Butt *et al.*, 2013).

Clove (*Syzygiuma romaticum*)

Cloves are the dried flower buds obtained from Syzygiumaromaticum tree. Clove possesses anti-inflammatory, antidiabetic, anesthetic, pain-relieving, antithrombotic and insect-repellent properties. The main ingredients found in clove are eugenol (50-87%), eugenyl acetate, tanene, thymol, and b-cariophyllene. These components are responsible for clove extract's effect when used under different conditions. In addition, these components have been shown to modulate some immune responses, including anti-inflammatory effects (Dibazar, 2014).The components also exhibit antimicrobial, anti-fungal, and anti-viral properties, and also possesses anti-inflammatory, cytotoxic, and anesthetic properties. Researchers found that the constituents of clove impart anti-oxidant activities and inhibit lipid peroxidation (Chaieb *et al.,* 2007).

CONCLUSION

The COVID-19 pandemic has claimed many lives and people with lower immunity are at more risk of getting coronavirus infection. In wake of this situation, boosting the immune system of body has gained worldwide attention. People are looking towards indigenous and traditional ways of boosting immunity. India is a hub of variety of medicinal herbs which are proved to have immunomodulating effects and thus can lessen the infection rate. Immunity cannot be built up in a day but intake of a well balanced diet and regular physical activity can keep the immune system in sound health.

This review focuses on the few Indian herbs like *Ashwagandha, Tulsi, Neem*, Garlic, Ginger, *Giloy* etc. in modulating and boosting immune system of our body. Intake of these herbs on a regular basis will result in a healthy immune system which in turn will help in combating this current pandemic.

REFERENCES

Arreola R, Quintero-Fabián S, López-Roa RI, Flores-Gutiérrez EO, Reyes-Grajeda JP, Carrera-Quintanar L, Ortuño-Sahagún D (2015) Immunomodulation and Anti-Inflammatory Effects ofGarlic Compounds. *J Immunol Res*, Special Issue.Volume 2015, Article ID 401630.

Aryaeian N, Tavakkoli H. (2015) Gingerand its effects on inflammatory diseases. *Adv Food Technol Nutr Sci Open* **1(4)**: 97-101.

Boroumand N, Samarghandian S, Hashemy SI (2018) Immunomodulatory, anti-inflammatory, and antioxidant effects of curcumin. *J Herbmed Pharmacol* **7(4)**: 211-219.

Butt MS, PashaI, Sultan MT, Randhawa MA, Saeed F, Ahmed W (2013) Black pepper and health claims: a comprehensive treatise *Crit Rev Food Sci Nutr* **53(9)**: 875-886.

Catanzaro M, Corsini E, Rosini M, Racchi M, Lanni C (2018) Immunomodulators Inspired by Nature: A Review on Curcumin and Echinacea. *Molecules* **23(11)**: 2778.

Chaieb K, Hajlaoui H, Zamantar T (2007) The chemical composition and biological activity of clove essential oil, Eugenia caryophyllata (Syzugiumaromaticum L Myrtaceae): A short review. *Phytother Res* **21**: 501-506.

Chandra RK (2003) Nutrient regulation of immune functions.*Forum Nutr* **56**: 147-148.

Chowdhury MA, Hossain N, Kashem MA, Shahid MA, Alam A (2020) Immune response in COVID-19: A review. *J Infect Public Health*, https://doi.org/10.1016/j.jiph.2020.07.001.

Cohen M (2014) *Tulsi - Ocimum sanctum*: A herb for all reasons. *J Ayurveda Integr Med*, **5 (4):**251-259.

Davis L, Kuttan G (2000) Immunomodulatory activity of Withaniasomnifera. *J Ethnopharmacol* **71:** 193–200.

Dibazar SP, Fateh S, Daneshmandi S (2014) Clove (Syzygiumaromaticum) ingredients affect lymphocyte subtypes expansion and cytokine profile responses: An in vitro evaluation. *J Food Drug Anal* **22:** 448-454.

Felsenstein S, Herbert JA, McNamara PS, Hedrich CM (2020) COVID-19: Immunology and treatment options. *Clin Immunol* **215** 108448.doi.org/10.1016/j.clim.2020.108448

GiriRP, Gangawane AK, Giri SG (2019) *Neem* the Wonder Herb: A Short Review. *Int J Trend Sci Res Dev* **3(3):** 962-967.

Greiner T (2011) Vitamins and minerals for women: recent programs and intervention trials. *Nutr Res Pract* **5(1):**3-10.

Grover HS, Deswal H, Singh Y, Bhardwaj A. (2015) Therapeutic effects of *Amla* in medicine and dentistry: A review. *J Oral Res Rev* **7:** 65-68.

Gruenwald J, Freder J, Armbruester N (2010) Cinnamon and Health. *Crit Rev Food Sci Nutr* **50:** 822–834.

Jagetia GC, Aggarwal BB (2007) "Spicing Up" of the Immune System by Curcumin. *J Clin Immunol* **27(1):** 19-35.

Jana SN, Madhu Charan S (2018) Health Benefits and Medicinal Potency of Withaniasomnifera: A Review. *Int J Pharm Sci Rev Res* **48(1):** 22-29.

Karacabey K, Ozdemir N (2012) The Effect of Nutritional Elements on the Immune System. *J Obes Wt Loss Ther* **2(9):** 1-6.

Kussmann M (2010) Nutrition and Immunity. **In:** RSC Food Analysis Monographs No. 9. Mass Spectrometry and Nutrition Research. Edited by Laurent B. Fay and Martin Kussmann. The Royal Society of Chemistry, UK, pp. 268-300.

Madhuri S., Pandey G, Verma KS (2011) Antioxidant, immunomodulatory and anticancer activities of *Emblicaofficinalis*: An Overview. *Int Res J Pharm* **2(8):** 38-42.

Mashhad NS, Ghiasvand R, Askari G, Hariri M, DarvishiL, Mofid MR (2013) Anti-Oxidative and Anti-Inflammatory Effects of Ginger in Health and Physical Activity: Review of Current Evidence. *Int J Prev Med* **4(Suppl 1):** S36–S42.

Ministry of AYUSH (2020). Ayurveda's immunity boosting measures for self care during COVID 19 crisis. https://www.mohfw.gov.in/pdf/Immunity Boosting AYUSHA dvisory.pdf

Ministry of Health and Family Welfare, GOI (2020). Detail Question and Answers on COVID-19 for Public. https://www.mohfw.gov.in/pdf/FAQ.pdf

Momtazi-Borojeni AA, Haftcheshmeh SM, Esmaeili SA, Johnston TP, Abdollahi E, Sahebkar A. (2018) Curcumin: A natural modulator of immune cells in systemic lupus erythematosus. *Autoimmun Rev* **17**:125–135.

Mukherjee PK, Nema NK, Bhadra S, Mukherjee D, Braga FC, Matsabisa MG (2014) Immunomodulatory leads from medicinal plants. *Indian J Tradit Know* 13(2): 235-256.

National Health Portal, GOI (2020). Introduction and Importance of Medicinal Plants and Herbs.https://www.nhp.gov.in/introduction-and-importance-of-medicinal-plants-and-herbs_mtl.

Nilashi M, Sama S, Shahmoadi L, Ahmadi H, Akbari E, Rashid TA (2020) The COVID-19 infection and the immune system: The role of complementaryand alternative medicines. *Biomed Res* **31(2):** 1-4.

Panchabhai TS, Kulkarni UP, Rege NN (2008) Validation of therapeutic claims of Tinosporacordifolia: a review. *Phytother Res* **22(4):** 425-41.

Rawat N, Roushan R (2018) Guduchi: A Potential Drug **In:** Ayurveda *World J Pharm Res* **7(12):** 355-361.

Reifen R (2002) Vitamin A as an anti-inflammatory agent. *Proceedings of the Nutrition Society* **61:** 397–400.

Roussel AM, Hininger I, Benaraba R, Ziegenfuss TN, Anderson RA (2009) Antioxidant effects of a cinnamon extract in people with impaired fasting glucose that are overweight or obese. *J Am Coll Nutr* **28(1):** 16-21.

Sai Krishna G, BhavaniRameshT, PremKumarP (2014) *"Tulsi"*- the Wonder Herb (PharmacologicalActivities of Ocimum Sanctum) *Am J Ethno*, **1(1):** 089-095

Salman H, Bergman M, Bessler H, Punsky I, Djaldetti M (1999) Effect ofa garlic derivative (alliin) on peripheral blood cell immune responses. *Int J Immunopharmacol* **21(9):** 589-597.

Saxena C, Rawat G (2019) Tinosporacordifolia (*Giloy*) - Therapeutic Uses and Importance: A review. *Cur Res Pharm Sci* **9(03):** 42-45.

Shang A, Cao S, Xu XY, Gan RY, Tang GY, Corke H, Mavumengwana V, Li HB (2019) Bioactive Compounds and Biological Functions of Garlic (*Allium sativum* L.). *Foods* **8(7):** 246

Singletary KW (2010) Black Pepper: Overview of Health Benefits. *Nutr Today* **45(1):** 43-47.

SrivasukiKP (2012) Nutritional and Health Care Benefits Of *Amla*. *J Pharmacogn* **3(2):** 147-151.

Upadhyay RK (2017) *Tulsi*: A holy plant with high medicinal andtherapeuticvalue. *Int J Green Pharm* **11(1):** S1–S12.

Verma SK, Kumar A (2011) Therapeutic uses of *Withaniasomnifera* (*Ashwagandha*) with a note on withanolides and its pharmacological actions. *Asian J Pharm Clin Res* **4(Suppl 1):** 1-4.

World Health Organization (2020). Health topics/ Coronavirus/ Overview.https://www.who.int/health-topics/coronavirus#tab=tab_1

Yadav DK, Bharitkar YP, Chatterjee K, GhoshM, Mondal NB, Swarnakar S (2016) Importance of *Neem* Leaf: An insight into its role in combating diseases. *Indian J. Exp Biol* **54(11):** 708-718.

Zheng W, Wang SY (2001) Antioxidant activity and phenolic compounds in selected herbs. *J Agric Food Chem.* **49(5):** 165-170.

Immunity Boosting Functional Foods to Combat COVID-19, Pages: 75–90
Edited by: Apurba Giri
Copyright © 2021, Narendra Publishing House, Delhi, India

CHAPTER - 7

POTENTIAL BENEFITS OF BERRIES AND THEIR BIOACTIVE COMPOUNDS AS FUNCTIONAL FOOD COMPONENT AND IMMUNE BOOSTING FOOD

Ritika B. Yadav

*Assistant Professor, Department of Food Technology,
Maharshi Dayanand University, Rohtak-124001, Haryana, India
E-mail: rita.by@rediffmail.com*

ABSTRACT

In the current condition of spread of corona virus, one of the preventive methods is to improve the strength of the immune system by eating the immunity boosting fruits. Berry fruits such as cranberry, blackberry, blueberry, strawberry and raspberry are rich in bioactive compounds. The bioactive compounds like phenolic acids and flavonoids are of great interest of food technologists and nutritionists due to their health benefits and immunity enhancing property. The phenolic compounds are phenolic acids, flavonoids, stilbenes, lignans, and tannins. Studies revealed that all these bioactive compounds are antioxidants and are found to be helpful in prevention of various diseases like cardiovascular disorders, diabetes, obesity and cancer. Berries also contain a variety of other nutrients, such as vitamins, minerals, carotenoids, organic acids, and dietary fibers. Several studies have reported that berries have antioxidant, antimutagenic, anticarcinogenic and anti-proliferative properties. The berry extracts obtained from berry fruits are act as free radical inhibitors. The polyphenolic compounds present in the berry fruit are responsible for the free radical scavenging activity. The consumption of plant foods that are rich in flavonoids has been claimed to protect against certain cancers such as lung cancer, and cardiovascular disease. Berry extracts are also helpful in inhibition of LDL oxidation. The daily consumption of berry fruits has proved to significantly decrease the occurrence of cancer, heart disease, cardiac stroke, and other degenerative diseases caused by oxidative stress. Due to good health promoting benefits, berry phenolic compounds can be useful as a functional ingredient in food industry for preparation of new functional food products.

Keywords: Berry fruits, Bioactive compounds, Phenolics, Flavonoids, Health benefits, Industrial applications

INTRODUCTION

Berry fruits are the clusters of one-seeded drupelets and are called as aggregate fruits. There are different varieties of berry fruits that have been cultivated through the centuries. Berry fruits mainly consumed are blackberries *(Rubus fructicosus)*, blueberries (*Vaccinium corymbosum*), black raspberries (*Rubus occidentalis*), red raspberries (*Rubus idaeus*), cranberries (*Vaccinium macrocarpon*) and strawberries (*Fragaria X. ananassa*). Some "niche-cultivated" berries and wild berries, such as black currant, lingonberries, bilberries, and cloudberry, are also popular in some areas of the world (Seeram, 2008). Berries such as strawberry, blueberry, and raspberry are traditionally favourite desserts in all over the world. These are consumed not only in fresh forms but also used as processed food materials for yogurts, beverages, jam, and jellies (Seeram *et al.*, 2006).

Berries are rich in phytochemicals and nutrients and therefore, can protect the body from various disease and disorders. Berries contain many phenolic substances, which are good for human health. Phenolic substances are the major group of bioactive compounds and include flavonoids (flavanones, flavones, flavanols, flavonols, anthocyanins and isoflavonoids), tannins, stilbenes, and phenolic acids. These compounds have antimutagenic and anti-carcinogenic properties (Rice-Evans and Miller, 1998). Some berries like black raspberries and strawberries, have been reported as high in phenolics like ellagic and gallic acid, which have anticancer activity (Xue *et al.*, 2002). The other phenolic substances and anthocyanins have antioxidant activity, which is important for physiological function (Liu *et al.*, 2002; Moyer *et al.*, 2002; Wang and Mazza, 2002). Anthocyanidins and anthocyanins have various biological effects, for example, anti-carcinogenesis, anti-diabetes, apoptosis induction, and prevention of obesity (Sakakibara *et al.*, 2002; Katsube *et al.*, 2003; Sasaki *et al.*, 2007; Tsuda, 2008). The flavonoids, like quercentin, phloretin, and apigenin stop the proliferation of cancer cells through the apoptosis inducing action (Kunts *et al.*, 1999; Wang *et al.*, 1999; Iwashita *et al.*, 2000). The consumption of plant foods that are rich in flavonoids has been claimed to prevent certain cancers like lung cancer, and cardiovascular disease (Hollman and Arts, 2005).

Epidemiological evidence revealed that high consumption of berries may provide protection against coronary heart disease, smoke and lung cancer (Hertog *et al.*, 1993, Keli *et al.*, 1996, Knekt *et al.*, 1997). In an earlier study, phenolic compounds from berry extracts inhibited the low-density lipoprotein (LDL) and oxidation of liposome (Heinonen *et al.*, 1998). Some studies reported that oxidation of low density lipoproteins (LDL) is related with cardiovascular disease (Mertens and Holvoet, 2001; Reed, 2002), and the flavonoid compounds due to their antioxidant activity are found to be linked with the protection from these diseases. Berry extracts play a significant role in inhibition of LDL oxidation in order: blackberries > red raspberries > blueberries > strawberries. In the same study, red raspberries, blueberries, strawberries and blackberries were also reported as inhibitor of oxidation of lecithin liposomes. The extracts obtained from raspberry, blackberry and gooseberry are act as free radical inhibitors (Heinonen and Meyer, 2000). Free radical scavenging capacity of berry fruit is due to the presence of their polyphenolic compounds. Small berries are good source of potential health promoting phytochemicals which are obtained from the *Ribes, Vaccinium, Ribus* and *Fragaria* genera. *Vaccinium* genera include cranberry, blueberry, and lingonberry. *Ribes* genera include red raspberries, blackberries and black raspberries. The gooseberry, currants are belonging to *Ribus* genera. Berry extracts are also used as dietary supplement for their good health benefits. Several studies have reported the antioxidant, anticancer, and anti-proliferative activity of berries (Meysken and Szabo, 2005; Seeram, 2006). This review describes the potential benefits of berry fruits and the bioactive compounds present in them as functional food component and immune boosting food.

General Composition and Bioactive Compounds

Berries are good source of bioactive compounds and most of which are phenolics. The phenolics include flavonoids and phenolic acids. Berries also contain a variety of other nutrients, such as vitamins, minerals (manganese, calcium, magnesium, iron and sodium), carotenoids, organic acids (malic acid, citric acid, tartaric, fumaric acid and oxalic acid) and dietary fibers. Berries are rich in pro-vitamin A, vitamin B, folic acid and vitamin C. These vitamins play an important role to improve the strength of the immune system and also lessen the inflammation. Berries are rich in ascorbic acid which acts as an antioxidant and helpful in scavenging the free radicals. Berry fruits have approximate 15% soluble solids which mainly consist of sugars. The main sugars in berries are fructose, glucose, and sucrose. However, the amount of sugar varies among cultivars. The good amount of fructose makes them useful for diabetic persons. The dietary fiber is also significant as it acts as intestinal regulator (Ramadan *et al.*, 2008).

Phenolic Compounds

Berry fruits are rich in phenolic compound which work as an antioxidant that are beneficial for human health. Phenolic compounds are a major group of bioactive compounds in berries including flavonoids, stibenes, hydrolysable tannins and simple phenolic acids (Fig.1) (Herken and Guzel, 2010). High intake of berries has been associated to the protection from degenerative disorders, like cardiovascular disease, cancer, diabetes, and arthritis (Adnan *et al.*, 2011). The phenolic compounds of berries are very important because of their health promoting properties. Phenolic compounds works as antitumor, antioxidant and anti-carcinogenic agents (Raspisarda *et al.*, 1999).

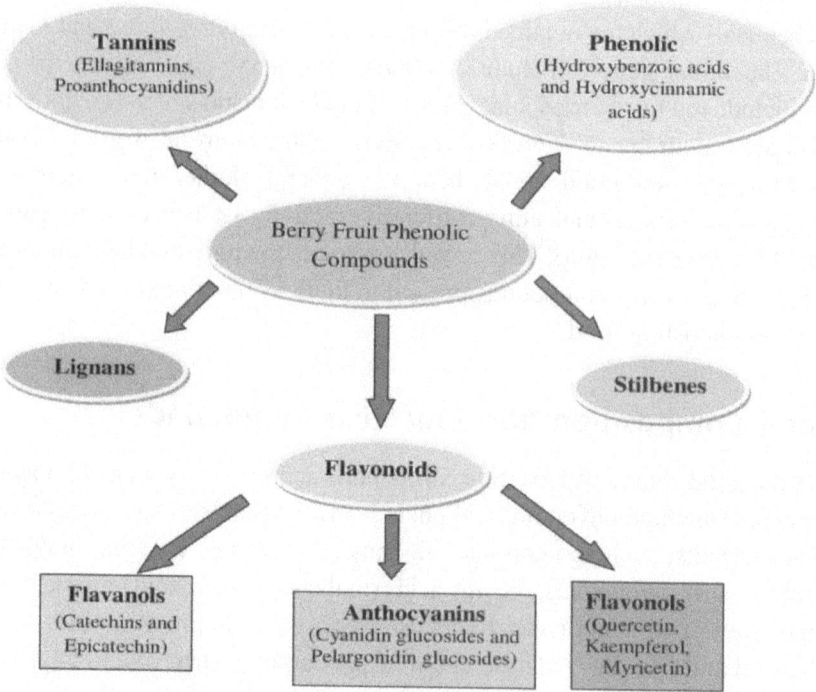

Fig. 1. Bioactive compounds in berry fruits

Flavonoids

Flavonoids are the second major group of bioactive compounds in berries including anthocyanins, flavanols and flavonols. Anthocyanins are the coloured pigments and gives especially red, blue, and purple colur to berries. The anthocyanins are linked with low risk of cancers, urinary tract health, improved aging, and memory. Juice, jam, wine, and food colorants prepared from berry fruits also contribute significantly to the intake of anthocyanins (Lopes *et al.*, 2007). The flavanols are another major phytochemical present in berries. The flavanols include catechin, epicatechin, gallocatechin, and epigallcatechin. Flavonols include myricetin, quercetin, and kaempferol. Quercetin has great health promoting effect as a cold and flu remedy, as anti-rheumatic and diuretic. Berry flavonoids have good anticarcogenic, antioxidant, anti-inflammatory and antimicrobial properties.

Types of Berries

There are several types of berry fruits which are as follow:

Cranberry

Cranberry (*Vaccinium macrocarpon*) is a member of family Ericaceae. The fruits are small in size and dark red in color that are native from eastern North America (Winston *et al.*, 2002). Common name of cranberries are American cranberry, large cranberry and in India cranberry known as *karaunda*. Cranberries are a good source of antioxidant flavonoids and phytochemicals. Cranberries are beneficial for immune and cardiovascular systems and, also have anticancer properties (Zhang and Zuo, 2004; Seifried *et al.*, 2007).

Strawberry

The strawberry (*Fragaria ananassa*) belongs to the family *Rosaceae*. Common name of strawberry are wild Indian strawberry or mock strawberry and in Hindi it is called as *hisalu* or *kiphaliya* in India. Strawberries are mostly eaten as fresh fruit and also used in processed food products like jam, preserves, ice creams and yogurts. Strawberry has anticancer, antioxidant, anti-proliferative, anti-inflammatory and anti-neurodegenerative activities (Hannum, 2004).

Blackberry

Blackberries (*Rubus fruticosus* sp.) also relate to family *Rosaceae*. The common name of blackberry is *Jamun*. Blackberries are rich in antioxidants and anthocyanins (Halvorsen *et al.*, 2006; Pantelidis *et al.*, 2007). The range of total phenolic and anthocyanin contents of blackberries have been reported to be 1.73-3.79 and 0.95-1.97 mg/g, respectively (Koca and Karadeniz, 2009).

Raspberry

The raspberries belong to the family *Rosaceae* and genus *Rubus* and the subgenus *idaeobatus*. Common name of raspberries are ceylon blackberry, cheeseberry, *Himalayan* raspberry and the local name is yellow raspberry and in Hindi name is *rasbhari*. Raspberries are high in phenolic acids, anthocyanin, and some other flavonoids (Mullen *et al.*, 2002). Raspberries contain high amount of vitamins and minerals (Wang and Lin, 2000).

Chokeberry

Chokeberries (*Aronia melanocarpa*) relate to the *Rosaceae* family. The common names of chokeberry are wild cherry, wild blackberry, bird cherry and bitter berry. Chokeberries are good source of polyphenols, mostly anthocyanins and procyanidins (Wu *et al.*, 2004). The extract of chokeberries exhibits the anti-proliferative and anti-carcinogenic activities (Bermudez-soto *et al.*, 2007).

Blueberry

The blueberries belong to the family *Ericaceae* and the genus *Vaccinium*. The common name of blueberry is jamun. Blueberries are high in bioactive compounds like phenolic acids, anthocyanins, flavonols (quercetin, kaempferol, and myricetin), ascorbic acid and flavanols (catechin, and epicatechin).

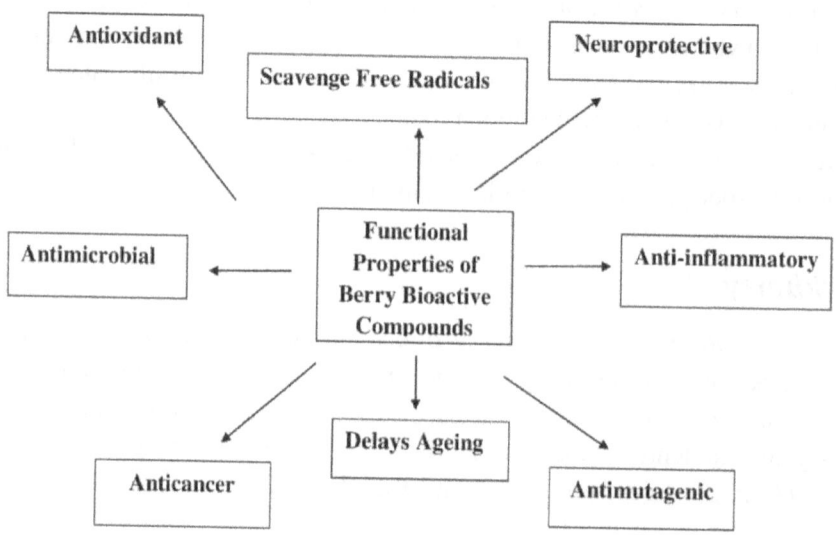

Fig. 2. Functional properties of berry bioactive compounds

Potential Health Benefits

Berries are rich in many naturally occurring antioxidants, like phenolic acids, flavonoids, vitamin C and vitamin E. Bioactive compounds and functional properties of berries are given in Table 1. They have health promoting effect including antioxidant, anticancer, and anti-inflammatory properties (Fig. 2). The berries also have the free radicals scavenging effect and protect the body from various types of cancers. Some berry fruits like strawberries, blueberries, and cranberries are rich in vitamin C which is useful for growth of strong connective tissues and gives strength to the immune system of the body. The berry leaves and fruits can also be helpful to relieve sore throats, nausea, sore mouths, diabetes, diarrhoea, inflammation, and dysentery (Schieber et al., 2001; WHO, 2002). Phytochemical present in berries are found to be helpful in lowering the risk of heart disorders, cancer, and delay of aging. Berry fruits are high in antioxidants such as vitamin E, vitamin C and anthocyanins that are helpful in protection of body against the damaging effect caused by free radicals. Table 2 shows the functional properties and mechanism of action of bioactive compounds of berries. Bioactive compounds of berries also have anticancer effects by various mechanisms like the induction of metabolizing enzymes, modulation of gene expression, induce apoptosis, and inhibit the cell proliferation. Shin et al. (2007) stated that the strawberry extract is helpful to stop the human liver cancer cell proliferation by 80%. The combined effect of phenolics and ascorbic acid of blueberries could stop the development of liver cancer cell and induce apoptosis (Yi et al., 2005). The extracts of berry fruits also possess anti-mutagenic activity and have an important role in inactivation of free radicals and inhibition of mutagenesis. The phytochemicals of berry fruits also have anti-inflammatory and anti-atherosclerotic effect which may protect the body against cardiovascular diseases (Meyer et al., 1998). Several authors also reported the anti-microbial activity of berry extracts (Kontiokari et al., 2003; Howell et al., 2005). Berry ellagitannins are strong anti-microbial agents and play a major role in prevention of colonization and infection of many pathogens (Puupponen-Pimia et al., 2005). Berries also provide other health benefits like prevention of obesity, diabetes and lipid disorders. Kowalska et al. (2017) reported the beneficial effect of extracts of chokeberry, bilberry, cranberry and raspberry in prevention of obesity through inhibition of adipogenesis and lipid accumulation.

Industrial Applications of Berries

Berries like blueberry, blackberry, raspberry, cranberry and strawberry are rich in bioactive compounds like phenolics and flavonoids and generally consumed as raw in fresh form. Berries are processed into jam, jellies, purees and desserts due

Table 1. Bioactive compounds and functional properties of berries

Berries	Bioactive Compounds	Functional Properties	References
Cranberry	Good source of vitamins C, calcium, magnesium iron and folate, quercetin, ellagic acid	Anticancer, antimutagenic or antitumorigenic, antibacterial, diuretic, reduction of the cardio-vascular disease, aids digestion, removes fats from lymphatic system	Bodet *et al.* (2008); Pappas and Schaich (2009)
Strawberry	High in vitamin C, quercetin, ellagic acid, anthocyanins (cyanidin-3-glucoside, pelargonidin, and pelargonidin-3-rutinoside)	Antioxidant, anti-proliferative, anticancer, diuretic, antioxidant, anti-diabetic, anti-inflammatory, reduce the occurrence of cardio-vascular disorders	Pinto Mda *et al.* (2010); Giampieri *et al.* (2015)
Blackberry	High in vitamin C, antioxidants, manganese, folate, polyphenols, ellagic acid and its glycosides, Cyanidin glycosides.	Antimicrobial, anti-inflammatory, scavenge free radical; antiseptic, inhibit colon tumor cell growth, reduces cholesterol, delays aging, neuroprotective	Jiao and Wang (2000); Siriwoharn *et al.* (2006)
Raspberry	High in vitamins C, gallic acid, ellagic acid, *p*-coumaric acid, caffeic acid, coumaroyl glyco-sides, antioxidants, folate, iron, copper, and lutein.	Anticancer; stop the growth of prostate, colon, oral and breast cancer cells, prevents free radical damage, antimicrobial and increases metabolic rate, which burns fats. good for eye health and strength.	Pantelidis *et al.* (2007); Szajdek and Borowska (2008)
Blueberry	High in vitamin C, zinc, iron, manganese, zea-xanthin and lutein, anthocyanins like cyanidine 3-glucoside, peonidin 3-glucoside and delphinidin.	Improve oxygen and blood supply to the eye, prevents free radical damage, good in bone protection, reduce the risk of cardiovascular disorders and prevention of atherosclerosis, anti-inflammatory, anti-diabetic, delays aging	Martineau, *et al.*, (2006); Shen *et al.* (2012); Calò and Marabini (2014)

Table 2. Functional properties and mechanism of action of bioactive compounds of berries

Functional properties	Mechanism of action	References
Antioxidant	Neutralization of free radicals, reduce the possibility of cardiovascular disorders by inhibiting the oxidation of LDL-cholesterol, or better vascular endothelial function, reduce the chance of occurrence of thrombosis	Basu, et al. (2010); Prasath, and Subramanian (2014)
Anticancer	Induction of metabolizing enzymes, regulation of gene expression, suppress the growth of cancer cells, and apoptosis inducing	Schantz et al. (2010); Liu et al. (2010); Srivastava et al. (2007)
Antimicrobial	Destabilization of cell membrane, permeabilization of plasma membrane, inhibition of extracellular microbial enzymes, and decrease microbial metabolic process.Berry ellagitannins are strong antimicrobial agents acting as possible anti-adherence compounds in preventing the colonization and infection of many pathogens	Puupponen-Pimia et al. (2005)
Neuroprotective	Increase serum antioxidant status, which is associated with low risk of degenerative and chronic diseases, improves hippocampal neurons survival and inhibits the pyramidal cell layer damage and increased SOD activity and decreased the MDA content in brain tissues and plasma in SAMP8 mice	Joseph et al. (2003); Tan et al. (2014)
Anti-inflammatory	Modulate enzyme activity, cellular pathways, and gene expression. Reducing oxidized-LDL formation via their antioxidant activity, Effective in reducing vascular endothelial growth factor expression, A promoter of angiogenesis, which is a critical step for tumor metastasis	Meyer et al. (1998); Liu et al. (2005); Ross et al. (2007)
Antimutagenic	Possess antimutagenic activity, which block cancer cell metabolism or kill cancer cells in culture, inactivate free radicals and active oxygen species, exhibit antiestrogenic activity, and inhibit mutagenesis inhibit the activity of the matrix metalloproteinases 2 and 9 involved in the invasion and metastasis of cancer cells.	Surh et al. (2001); Katsube et al. (2003)

to their seasonal nature. Berry fruits are also used in production of functional and nutraceutical foods. The value added products such as frozen, freeze-dried and vacuum-dried products from berries also have been developed. Bauman *et al.* (2006) described the method of vacuum puffed and expanded fruits including blueberries. Chokeberry contains highest amount of polyphenol content in comparison to other berries. This berry is mainly used in juices and only 10% is used for cosmetic products, diet supplements and fruit tea. The fresh juice from strawberries has higher anthocyanin, total phenolic content (TPC), and proanthocyanidin content in comparison to the stored one (Oszmiañski and Wojdy³o, 2009). Berries are also found wide applications in bakery products, fruit fillings, muffins, and canned forms. The berry fruits are rich in anthocyanins and therefore, they are used in production of food dyes (Skrovankova *et al.*, 2015; Kowalska *et al.*, 2017). Bioactive compounds present in berries also have wide applications as natural antimicrobial agents in the pharmaceuticals and food industries.

CONCLUSION

Berries constitute an important and significant source of bioactive compounds like flavonoids and phenolic acids which have good health promoting effects. The phenolic compounds and anthocyanins have antioxidant activity and helpful in scavenging the free radicals. Berries also contain some other nutrients like vitamins, minerals, carotenoids, organic acids, and dietary fibers. The bioactive compounds present in berries have many health-promoting effects including antioxidant, anticancer, anti-atherosclerotic, anti-inflammatory and anti-microbial properties. Bioactive compounds of berries also play a major role in delay of aging process. The functional and nutraceutical food could be developed using extracts from berry fruits due to their health benefits. The utilization of anti-microbial activity of bioactive compounds of berries also offers opportunities for their use in food industries as natural anti- microbial agents.

REFERENCES

Adnan L, Osman A, Hamid AA (2011) Antioxidant activity of different extracts of red pitaya (Hylocereus polyrhizus) seed. *Int J Food Prop* **14:** 1171-1181.

Basu A, Rhone M, Lyons TJ (2010) Berries: Emerging impact on cardiovascular health. *Nutr Rev* **68:** 168–177.

Bauman MN, Roy P, Sinha NK, Sinha M (2006) Vacuum puffed and expanded fruit. U.S. Published Patent Application No: 0013925AI.

Bermudez-Soto MJ, Larrosa M, Garcia-Cantalejo JM, Espin JC, Tomas- Barberan FA, Garcia- Conesa MT (2007) Up- regulation of tumor suppressor carcinoembryonic antigen related cell adhesion molecule 1 in human colon cancer caco-2 cells fallowing repetitive exposure to dietary levels of a polyphenol rich Chokeberry juice. *J Nutr Biochem* **18**: 259-71.

Bodet C, Grenire D, Chandad F, Ofek I, Steinberg D, Weiss E (2008) Potential oral health benefits of cranberry. *Crit Rev Food Sci Nutr* **48**: 672–80.

Calò R, Marabini L (2014) Protective effect of Vaccinium myrtillus extract against UVA- and UVB-induced damage in a human keratinocyte cell line (HaCaT cells). *J Photochem Photobiol Biol* **132**: 27–35.

Giampieri F, Forbes-Hernandez TY, Gasparrini M, Alvarez-Suarez JM, Afrin S, Bompadre S, Quiles JL, Mezzetti B, Battino M (2015) Strawberry as a health promoter: An evidence based review. *Food Funct* **6**: 1386–1398.

Halvorsen BL, Carlsen MH, Phillips KM, Bohn SK, Holte K, Jacobs DR (2006). Content of redox-active compounds in foods consumed in the United State. *Am J Clin Nutr* **84**: 95-135.

Hannum SM (2004) Potential impact of strawberries on human health. *Crit Rev Food Sci Nutr* **44**: 1-7.

Heinonen IM, Meyer AS (2000) Antioxidant in fruits, berries and vegetable. **In:** Fruit and vegetable processing improving quality, Ed. Jongen W, Woodhead Publishing Ltd., Cambridge, pp 23-51.

Heinonon IM, Meyer AS, Frankel EN (1998) Antioxidant activity of berry phenolics on cancer, low-density lipoprotein and liposome oxidation. *J Agric Food Chem* **46**: 4107-12.

Herken EN, Guzel S (2010) Total antioxidant capacity and total phenol contents of selected commercial fruit juices. *Croatian J Food Sci Tech* **1**: 9-17.

Hertog MGL, Hollman PCH, Van de Putte B (1993) Content of potentially anticarcinogenic flavonoids of tea infusions, wines, and fruit juices. *J Agric Food Chem* **41(8)**: 1242-1246.

Hollman PC and Arts IC (2005). Polyphenols and disease risk in epidemiologic studies. *Am J Clin Nutr* **81**: 317S- 325S.

Howell AB, Reed JD, Krueger CG, Winterbottom R, Cunningham DG, Leahy M (2005) A type cranberry proanthocyanidins and uropathogenic bacterial anti-adhesion activity. *J Phytochem* **66**: 2281–2291.

Iwashita M, Kobori M, Yamaki K, Tsushida T (2000). Flavonoids inhibit cell growth and induce apoptosis in B16 melanoma 4A5. *Biosci Biotechnol Biochem* **64**: 1813-1820.

Jiao H, Wang SY (2000) Correlation of antioxidant capacities to oxygen radical scavenging enzyme activities in blackberry. *J Agric Food Chem* **48**: 5672–6.

Joseph JA, Denisova NA, Arendash G, Gordon M, Diamond D, Shukitt-Hale B, Morgan D (2003) Blueberry supplementation enhancing signalling and prevents behavioural deficits in an Alzheimer disease model. *Nutr Neurosci* **6**: 153-162

Katsube N, Iwashita K, Tsushida T, Yamaki K, Kobori M (2003). Induction of apoptosis in cancer cells by bilberry (Vaccinium myrtillus) and the anthocyanins. *J Agric Food Chem* **51**: 68–75.

Keli SO, Hertog MGL, Feskens EJM, Kromhout D (1996) Dietary flavonoids, antioxidant vitamins, and incidence of stroke: the Zutphen study. *Arch Intern Med* **156**: 637-642.

Knekt P, Jarvinen R, Seppanen R, Hellovaara M, Teppo L, Pukkala E, Aromaa A (1997) Dietary flavonoids and the risk of lung cancer and other malignant neoplasms. *Am J Epidemiol* **146**: 223-230.

Koca I, Karadeniz B (2009) Antioxidant properties of blackberry and blueberry fruits grown in the Black Sea region of Turkey. *Scientia Horticultural* **121**: 447-50.

Kontiokari T, Laitinen J, Jrvi L, Pokka T, Sundqvist K, Uhari M (2003) Dietary factors protecting women from urinary tract infections. *Am J Clin Nutr* **77**: 600–604.

Kowalska, K, Olejnik A, Szwajgier D, Olkowicz M (2017) Inhibitory activity of chokeberry, bilberry, raspberry and cranberry polyphenol-rich extract towards adipogenesis and oxidative stress in differentiated 3T3-L1 adipose cells. *Plos One* **12(11)**, 1-15.

Kunts S, Wenzel U, Daniel H (1999). Comparative analysis of the effects of flavonoids on proliferation, cytotoxicity, and apoptosis in human colon cancer cell lines. *Eur J Nutr* **38**: 133-142.

Liu J, Zhang W, Jing H, Popovich DG (2010) Bog bilberry (*Vaccinium uliginosum* L.) extract reduces cultured Hep-G2, Caco-2, and 3T3-L1 cell viability, affects cell cycle progression, and has variable effects on membrane permeability. *J Food Sci* **75**: 103–107.

Liu M, Li XQ, Weber C, Lee CY, Brown J, Liu RH (2002) Antioxidant and antiproliferative activities of raspberries. *J. Agric. Food Chem* **50**: 2926-2930.

Liu Z, Schwimer J, Liu D, Greenway FL, Anthony CT, Woltering EA (2005) Black raspberry extract and fractions contain angiogenesis inhibitors. *J Agric Food Chem* **53**: 3909–3915.

Lopes da-Silva F, Escribano-Bailon MT, Perez-Alonso JJ, Rivas-Gonzalo J, Santos-Buelga C, (2007) Anthocyanin pigments in strawberry. *LWT Food Sci Technol* **40**: 374–82.

Martineau LC, Couture A, Spoor D, Benhaddou-Andaloussi A, Harris C, Meddah B, Leduca C, Burtc A, Vuonga T, Le PM *et al.* (2006) Anti-diabetic properties of the Canadian lowbush blueberry *Vaccinium angustifolium* Ait. *Phytomed* **13**: 612–623.

Mertens A, Holvoet P (2001) Oxidized LDL and HDL: Antagonists in atherothrombosis. *FASEB J* **15**: 2073-2084.

Meyer AS, Heinonen M, Frankel EN (1998) Antioxidant interactions of catechin cyaniding caffeic acid quercetin and ellagic acid on human LDL oxidation. *Food Chem* **61**: 71–75.

Meyskens FL, Szabo E (2005) Diet and cancer: the disconnect between epidemiology and randomized clinical trials. *Cancer Epidem Biomar Prev* **14**: 1366–9.

Moyer RA, Hummer KM, Finn CE, Frei B, Wrolstad RE (2002) Anthocyanins, phenolics, and antioxidant capacity in diverse small fruits: Vaccinium, Rubus, and Ribes. *J Agric Food Chem* **50**: 519-525.

Mullen W, Mc-Ginn J, Lean MEJ, MacLean MR, Gardner P, Duthie GG, Yokota T (2000) Ellagitannins, flavonoids and other phenolics in red raspberries and their contribution to antioxidant capacity and vasorelaxation properties. *J Agric Food Chem* **50**: 5191-5196.

Oszmiañski J, Wojdy³o A (2009) Comparative study of phenolic content and antioxidant activity of strawberry puree, clear, and cloudy juices. *Eur Food Res Technol* **228**: 623–631.

Pantelidis GE, Vasilakakis M, Manganaris GA, Diamantidis G (2007) Antioxidant capacity, phenol, anthocyanins and ascorbic acid contents in raspberries, blackberries, red currants, gooseberries and cornelian cherries. *Food Chem* **102**: 777-783.

Pappas E, Schaich M (2009) Phytochemicals of cranberries and cranberry products characterization potential health effects and processing stability. *Crit Rev Food Sci Nutr* **49**: 741–81.

Pinto Mda S, de Carvalho JE, Lajolo FM, Genovese MI, Shetty K (2010) Evaluation of antiproliferative, anti-type 2 diabetes, and antihypertension potentials of ellagitannins from strawberries (Fragaria ananassa Duch.) using in vitro models. *J Med Food* **13:** 1–9.

Prasath GS, Subramanian SP (2014) Antihyperlipidemic effect of fisetin, a bioflavonoid of strawberries, studied in streptozotocin-induced diabetic rats. *J Biochem Mol Toxicol* **28:** 442–449.

Puupponen-Pimia R, Nohynek L, Hartmann-Schmidlin S, Kahkonen M, Heinonen M, Maastta-Riihinen K (2005). Berry phenolics selectively inhibit the growth of intestinal pathogens. *J Appl Microbiol* **98:** 991–1000.

Ramadan MF, Sitohy MZ, Morsel JT (2008) Solvent and enzyme-aided aqueous extraction of goldenberry (Physalis peruviana L) pomace oil impact of processing on composition and quality of oil and meal. *Eur J Food Res Technol* **226:** 1445–1448.

Rapisarda P, Tomaino A, Lo Cascio R, Bonina F, De Pasquale A, Saija A (1999) Antioxidant effectiveness as influenced by phenolic content of fresh orange juices. *J Agric Food Chem* **47:** 4718-4723.

Reed J (2002) Cranberry flavonoids, atherosclerosis and cardiovascular health. *Crit Rev Food Sci Nutr* **42:** 301-316.

Rice-Evans CA, Miller NJ (1998) Structure-antioxidant activity relationships of flavonoids and isoflavonoids. **In:** Flavonoids in health and disease Rice-Evans CA, Packer C, (ed.), Marcel Dekker New York, pp. 199-219.

Ross HA, McDougall GJ, Stewart D (2007) Antiproliferative activity is predominantly associated with ellagitannins in raspberry extracts. *Phytochem* **68:** 218–228.

Sakakibara H, Ashida H, Kanazawa K (2002) A novel method using 8-hydroperoxy-22 -deoxyguanosine formation for evaluating antioxidative potency. *Free Radic Res J* **36:** 307–316.

Sasaki R, Nishimura N, Hoshino H, Isa Y, Kadowaki M, Ichi T, Tanaka A, Nishiumi S, Fukuda I, Ashida H, Horio F, Tsuda T (2007) Cyanidin 3-glucoside ameliorates hyperglycemia and insulin sensitivity due to downregulation of retinol binding protein 4 expression in diabetic mice. *J Biochem Pharmacol* **74:** 1619–1627.

Schantz M, Mohn C, Baum M, Richling E (2010) Antioxidative efficiency of an anthocyanin rich bilberry extract in the human colon tumor cell lines Caco-2 and HT-29. *J Berry Res* **1:** 25–33.

Schieber A, Stintzing FC, and Carle R. (2001) By-products of plant food processing as a source of functional compounds- recent developments. *J Food Sci Technol* **12:** 401–13.

Seeram NP (2006) Berries. **In:** Nutritional oncology. Heber D, Blackburn G, Go VLW, Milner J (ed), 2nd edn. London, UK, Academic Press pp. 615–25.

Seeram PN (2008) Berry fruits: compositional elements, biochemical activities, and the impact of their intake on human health, performance, and disease. *J Agric Food Chem* **56:** 627–629.

Seeram PN, Adams SL, Zhao Y, Lee R, Sand D, Scheuller SH, Heber D (2006) Blackberry, black raspberry, blueberry, cranberry, red raspberry, and strawberry extracts inhibit growth and stimulate apoptosis of human cancer cells in vitro. *J Agric Food Chem* **54:** 9329–9339.

Seifried HE, Anderson DE, Fisher EI, Milner JA (2007) A review of the interaction among dietary antioxidants and reactive oxygen species. *J Nutr Biochem* **18:** 567-79.

Shen, CL, von Bergen V, Chyu MC, Jenkins MR, Mo H, Chen C-H (2012) Kwun IS fruits and dietary phytochemicals in bone protection. *Nutr Res* **32:** 897–910.

Shin Y, Liu RH, Nock JF, Holliday D, Watkins CB (2007) Temperature and relative effects on quality, total ascorbic acid, phenolics and flavonoids concentration and antioxidase on strawberry. *Postharvest Biol Technol* **45:** 349-357.

Siriwoharn T, Wrolstad RE, Durst RW (2006) Identification of ellagic acid in blackberry juice sediment. *J Food Sci* **70:** 189–97.

Skrovankova S, Sumczynski D, Mlcek J, Jurikova T, Sochor J (2015). Bioactive compounds and antioxidant activity in different types of berries. *Int J Mol Sci 16:* 24673-24706.

Srivastava A, Akoh CC, Fischer J, Krewer G (2007) Effect of anthocyanin fractions from selected cultivars of Georgia-grown blueberries on apoptosis and phase II enzymes. *J Agric Food Chem* **55:** 3180–3185.

Surh YJ, Na HK, Lee JY, Keum YS (2001) Molecular mechanisms underlying antitumor promoting activities of heat-processed Panax ginseng CA Meyer. *J Korean Med Sci* **16:** S38–41.

Szajdek A, Borowska JE (2008) Bioactive compounds and health-promoting properties of berry fruits a review. *Plant Foods Hum Nutr* **63:** 147–56.

Tan L, Yang HP, Pang W, Lu H, Hu YD, Li J, Lu SJ, Zhang WQ, Jiang YG (2014) Cyanidin-3-O-galactoside and blueberry extracts supplementation improves spatial memory and regulates hippocampal ERK expression in senescence-accelerated mice. *Biomed Environ Sci* **27(3):** 186-196.

Tsuda T (2008) Regulation of adipocyte function by anthocyanins, possibility of preventing the metabolic syndrome. *J. Agric. Food Chem* **56**: 642-646.

Wang IK, Lin-Shiau SY, Lin JK (1999) Induction of apoptosis by apigenin and related flavonoids through cytochrome c release and activation of caspase-9 and caspase-3 in leukemia HL-60 cells. *Eur J Cancer* **35**: 1517-1525.

Wang J, Mazza G (2002) Inhibitory effects of anthocyanins and other phenolic compounds on nitric oxide production in LPS/IFN-ç-activated RAW 264.7 macrophages. *J Agric Food Chem* **50**: 850-857.

Wang S, Lin HS (2000) Antioxidant activity in fruits and leaves of blackberry, raspberry and strawberry varieties with cultivar and developmental stage. *J Agric Food Chem* **18**: 140–146.

WHO (2002) The World Health Report Reducing risks and promoting healthy life. Geneva, Switzerland: World Health Organization.

Winston D, Graff A, Brinckman J, Langer R, Turner A, Reich E, Bieber A, Howell A, Romm A (2002) Cranberry fruit, Vaccinium macrocarpon aiton. **In:** Standards of Analysis, Quality Control, and Therapeutics ed. Upton R, Graff A Santa Cruz CA: American Herbal Pharmacopoeia and Therapeutic compendium, American Herbal Pharmacopoeia.

Wu X, Gu L, Prior RL, McKay S (2004). Characterization of anthocyanins and proanthocyanidins in some cultivars of Ribers, Aronia and Sambucus and their antioxidant capacity. *J Agric Food Chem* **52**: 7846-56.

Xue H, Aziz RM, Sun N, Cassady JM, Kamendulis LM, Xu Y (2002) Inhibition of cellular transformation by berry extracts. *Carcinog* **22**: 351–356.

Yi W, Fischer J, Krewer G, Akoh CC (2005) Phenolic compounds from blueberries can inhibit colon cancer cell profiferation and induce apoptosis. *J Agric Food Chem* **53**: 7320–7329.

Zhang K, Zuo Y (2004) GC-MS determination of flavonoids and phenolic and benzoic acids in human plasma after consumption of cranberry juice. *J Agric Food Chem* **52**: 222-227.

Immunity Boosting Functional Foods to Combat COVID-19, Pages: 91–101
Edited by: Apurba Giri
Copyright © 2021, Narendra Publishing House, Delhi, India

CHAPTER - 8

EFFECTIVENESS OF FLAX SEED, AN IMMUNE BOOSTER FUNCTIONAL FOOD DURING COVID-19 PANDEMIC SITUATION

Pritha Ghosh[1] and Subhadeep Dutta[2*]

[1]*M. Sc. in Applied Nutrition, National Institute of Nutrition, Indian Council of Medical Research, Hyderabad-500007, India*
E-mail: pritha.ratanpur@gmail.com
[2]*State Aided College Teacher, Department of Nutrition, Vivekananda Mahavidyalaya, Haripal-712405, West Bengal, India*
E-mail: subhadeepdutta@vmharipal.ac.in
*Corresponding author

ABSTRACT

During current COVID- 19 pandemic situation where preventive and curative medicines are unavailable, strong immune system is one of the best weapons to deal with it at individual level. Functional foods and dietary modification can decrease any kind of infections (viral as well as other infections) risk including COVID-19 and build up our immunity. Persons with strong immunity are able to recover any infectious disease conditions within short period of time. Main concern of this content is to support the principle that flax seed, a plant-derived omega-3 (ù-3) polyunsaturated fatty acids (rich in α-linolenic acid) can activate both adaptive and innate immune functions, altered macrophage function through production and secretion of cytokines and chemokines, improve phagocytosis capacity leads to increase immunity. Two bioactive compounds lignans and fiber are also present in flax seed. Flax seed reduces inflammation oxidative stress, and shows lipid modulating properties also. Omega -3 fatty acids popular for its health benefits against comorbidities in the COVID-19 patients including hypertension, respiratory system disease and cardiovascular disease, diabetes, cancer. Flax seed helps to maintain intestinal environment, function and immunity through modulating the gut microbiota composition, improve intestinal wall integrity, production of short chain fatty acids (due to fermentation of flaxseed fiber by gut microbiota). However it is established that the inclusion of sufficient amount of flax seed as whole, powder, oil, or fortified form in our regular diet helps to boost immunity against infectious disease.

Keywords: Immune system, Flax seed, Omega-3 PUFA, Comorbidities, Gut immunity, Prebiotic.

INTRODUCTION

COVID- 19 pandemic which extended over the world is now main public health concern worldwide. Consequently public health emergency is essential to prevent spreading rate of novel corona virus (SARS-CoV-2). COVID-19 virus contains single-stranded RNA (+ssRNA) (Cascella *et al.*, 2020). SARS-CoV-2 transmitted through coughing and sneezing (respiratory droplets). COVID-19 virus mainly target respiratory system. This virus attached with angiotensin-converting enzyme 2 receptors by their spikes (glycoprotein) which shows higher affinity towards SARS-CoV-2. ACE- 2 receptors are widely present t in type II alveolar cells of lungs (Budhwar *et al.*, 2020). Incubation period of the virus is 0 to 24 days (Zhong *et al.*, 2020). Common symptoms are cough, fever, shortness of breath, sore throat and fatigue which lead to Acute Respiratory Distress Syndrome (ARDS), pneumonia, and multiple organ dysfunctions in severe conditions (Singhal, 2020). Patients with comorbidities like diabetes, hypertension, obesity, cardiovascular disease, chronic lung disease, chronic kidney disease patients and cancer patients are at higher risk of infection (Sanyaolu *et al.*, 2020). Nutritional intervention is one of the effective ways to prevent any type of viral infection including COVID-19 and maintain immunity at the individual level. Negative nutrition status can increase the infection rate, viral load, mortality rate and delayed recovery from infections (Naja and hamadeh, 2020). Maintaining hydration, positive nutritional status, and boost up immune system are some common strategies to prevent the infection progression rate during this pandemic situation (Derbyshire and Delange, 2020). Functional foods have some additional positive effects on human body with basic nutrition. Functional foods are effectively uses to treat metabolic disease, non-communicable diseases and infectious disease. Some common functional ingredients are polyunsaturated fatty acids (PUFAs), probiotics, prebiotics, synbiotics, phytosterols and antioxidants (Granato *et al.*, 2020). Recently flaxseed is widely popular as healthy plant based functional food. It can prevent chronic diseases, comorbidities and maintain immune system of human body. Flaxseed also known as linseed (*Linum usitatissimum*) is rich in protein (22%), lipids (~41%), carbohydrates (~29%), and other essential micronutrients. Flaxseed is the rich source of plant derived omega-3 fatty acids (PUFA= ~29% of total dietary fat). Among omega-3 fatty acids, α-linolenic acid (ALA) is more abandoned that is near about 50%. All micro and macro nutrients present in flax seeds are generally recognized as safe (GRAS) and flaxseed itself consider as a 'superfood' for its various health benefits. High amount of lignans, fiber (cellulose, mucilage gums, and lignin) are also present in flaxseeds and have lots of health benefits (Christian *et al.*, 2018, Chiara *et al.*, 2020). Flaxseed commonly use as whole, milled, roasted and oil form (Goyal*et al.*, 2014). ALA in flaxseed oil is more bioavailable than milled flaxseed; again milled seed shows more bioavailability of ALA than whole flaxseed (Delfin *et al.*, 2010). Omega-3 PUFAs present in flaxseeds are used to improve immunity against viral infections, manage the "cytokine storm and decrease IL-6 and IL-1β level in plasma (Szabó *et al.*, 2020). The omega-3 fatty acid is effective against type 2 diabetes, kidney disease, rheumatoid arthritis, high blood pressure, coronary heart disease, stroke, alzheimerdisease, cancers that are considered as comorbidities and can enhance the severity of COVID-19 infection condition (Katare *et al.*, 2012). Flaxseed shows positive impact towards gut immunity (Haidari *et al.*, 2020).

Effect of Flaxseed Derived Omega-3 Fatty Acids Against Viral Infections Including SARS-CoV-2

Flaxseed contains higher amount of polyunsaturated fatty acid, moderate amount of monounsaturated fat, and low amount of saturated fat (9 %). Flaxseed contains good amount of both soluble and insoluble dietary fiber (around 35–45 %) and lignans. We can use flaxseed as an immune boosting functional food due to its various nutritional and immune boosting properties (Kajla and Sharma, 2015; Butler and Barrientos, 2020). Flaxseed oil is one of the major plant sources of n-3 poly unsaturated fatty acids and more than 50% of the n-3 PUFA present as alpha-linolenic acid (ALA). Omega-3 fatty inhibitsPGE2 and NF-κB that leads to suppress inflammatory response. It can also activate MAPK and GPR120 to reduce inflammation (Messina *et al.*, 2020; Marginγ *et al.*, 2020). Cytokine storm due to damage of host tissue by innate immunity is very common during COVID-19 infection. This situation leads to further lung injury and respiratory failure (ARDS) that is the main cause of death after COVID-19 infection. Inflammation occurs during the infection period due to systemic inflammatory response which triggers the release of pro-inflammatory cytokines such as IFN-α, TNF-α, IL-1β, IFN-γ, IL-6, IL-18, IL-12, IL-33, TGFβ, etc.) and chemokines (CXCL9, CXCL10, etc). High amount of inflammatory markers such as ferritin, C reactive protein and IL-6 levels are also noticeable in bloodstream. Omega-3 fatty acids with antioxidants can effectively reduce inflammation and the cytokine storm through their conversion to specialized pro-resolving mediators which helps to improve oxygenation and decrease the duration of mechanical ventilation, intensive care unit (Farrah *et al.*, 2018; Abbas *et al.*, 2020; Calder, 2020; Horowitz and Freeman, 2020; Magro *et al.*, 2020; Shakoor *et al.*, 2020). Omega-3 PUFAs exhibits phagocytosis activity of macrophages, maintain macrophage based innate immunity and helps to reduce viral propagation (Kumar, 2019, Hirayama *et al.*, 2018). Devarshi *et al.* (2013) also showed that flaxseed oil and fish oil based diet decreased the expression of TNF-α, IL-6 and adipocyte fatty acid-binding proteins in livers of diabetic rats (Devarshi *et al.*, 2013). Zhu *et al.* (2020) experimented effect of dietary flaxseed oil (FO) rich in omega-3 (ù-3) polyunsaturated fatty acids on diabetic rats and showed significant reduction in interleukin (IL)-1β, tumor necrosis factor (TNF)-α, IL-6, IL-17A , fasting blood glucose (FBG), glycated hemoglobin, blood lipid, plasma lipopolysaccharide and suppressing inflammation also. Ren *et al.* (2016) conducted a meta-analysis and proved the significant reduction of C- reactive protein in obese populations after consumption of flax seeds and its derivatives. Zhang *et al.* (2020) stated that omega 3 PUFA (protectin D1) used to prepare antiviral drug, an effective intervention for this novel virus, COVID 19. They also said that ALA might be an optional therapy for this novel virus.

Flaxseed to Boost Gut Immunity

Mammalian gastrointestinal tract is the largest immune organ in the body. Most of immune cells of the human body are found in gut-associated lymphoid tissue (GALT) (Childs *et al.*, 2019). Gastrointestinal tract gives protection against any kind of viral infection through intestinal epithelial cell barrier and regulating immune cell functions to decrease infection rate (Wu *et al.*, 2018). IgA secreted from subepithelial B-cells in the intestine shows many immune functions such as protection against enteropathogens, build up herd immunity towards enteropathogens, inhibitsantigen spreading into the circulation etc (Chassaing *et al.*, 2014). The gut microbiota can regulate the function of adaptive and the innateimmune system (Dhar and Mohanty, 2020). It also helps to maintain host defenses mechanisms against viral infections including respiratory viruses (He *et al.*, 2020, Van der Lelie and Taghavi, 2020). Gut microbiota diversity and beneficial microorganisms in the gut improves gut immune system which is another effective way to boost immunity against viral infections. Flaxseed contains a huge amount of lignans (75 to 800 times more than cereals) and fibers (both soluble and insoluble fiber) such as cellulose, hemicelluloses, mucilage gums, and lignin (Dzuvor *et al.*, 2018; Sanmartin *et al.*, 2020) which are known as prebiotics and helps to maintain good gut microbial environment (probiotics). Gut microbiota produce short-chain fatty acids (acetate, propionate, and butyrate) from dietary fibers which serve energy to colonocytes and enhance gut barrier integrity (Ndou *et al.*, 2018; Sherif *et al.*, 2019; Corona *et al.*, 2020). Some *in vivo* animal experiments also confirm that dietary flaxseed can effectively increase the production rate of SCFA by gut microbiota and exhibit the growth of healthy gut microbiota (Sherif *et al.*, 2019; Lili *et al.*, 2020).

Benefits of Flaxseed to the Patient with Comorbidities

Patients with comorbidities such as diabetes, chronic respiratory disease and cardiovascular diseases, HIV, liver disease, renal disease, asthma, hypertension, obesity, cancer are at the high risk of viral infection by COVID-19 virus (SARS-CoV-2) and also shows poorer clinical outcomes during treatment. Centers for Disease Control and Prevention and World Health organization also confirmed this statement (Ejaz *et al.*, 2020; Guan *et al.*, 2020; Yang *et al.*, 2020; Nogueira-de-Almeida *et al.*, 2020). Many clinical and experimental studies confirmed that flaxseed is very useful and effective to combat various cardiovascular diseases due to high content of α-Linolenic acid (ALA) (Rodriguez-Leyva *et al.*, 2010, Parikh *et al.*, 2018, Rogero *et al.*, 2020). Flaxseed can remarkably reduce lipid profiles (Triglycerides, total cholesterol, and low density lipoprotein) as well as anthropometric measurements (Waist circumference, Waist to hip ratio) of an individual (Haghighatsiar *et al.*, 2019). According to human and animal studies flaxseed supplementation significantly decreases both systolic and diastolic blood pressure (Stephanie *et al.*, 2014; Khalesi *et al.*, 2015; Ursoniu *et al.*, 2016) as well as showed benefits in diabetes (Thakur *et al.*, 2009; Hasaniani *et al.*, 2020; Jamilian *et al.*, 2020), and obesity (Mohammadi-Sartang *et al.*, 2017; Rezaei *et al.*, 2020) conditions.

CONCLUSION

During the COVID-19 pandemic situation it is very essential to boost our immune function against any kind of infections (viral as well as other infections). Improve immune functions through nutrition is one of the significant strategy during this uncertain time when appropriate drug or vaccine is not available to prevent this viral infection. However, it is proved that daily consumption of flaxseed can enhance and maintain the immune system of our body that are further helps to combat against viral and other infectious diseases through. It is long term process to increase our immunity through diet. Flaxseed and its derived products act as prebiotics, that can effectively maintain gut microbial composition and consequently improve gut Immunity. We can control and inhibit comorbidities related health risks also through flaxseed based diet. Improve immunity through diet is a long term process but most effective.

REFERENCES

Abbas AM, Kamel MM (2020) Dietary habits in adults during quarantine in the context of COVID-19 pandemic. *Obes Med* **19:** 100254.

Budhwar S, Sethi K, Chakraborty M (2020) A Rapid Advice Guideline for the Prevention of Novel Coronavirus through Nutritional Intervention. *CurrNutr Rep.* **9(3):** 119–128.

Butler M J, Barrientos RM (2020) The impact of nutrition on COVID-19 susceptibility and long-term consequences. *Brain Behav Immun* **87:** 53–54.

Calder PC (2020) Nutrition, immunity and COVID-19. *BMJ nutr. prev. health* doi: 10.1136/bmjnph-2020-000085.

Caligiuri SPB, Edel AL, Aliani M *et al* (2014) Flaxseed for Hypertension: Implications for Blood Pressure Regulation. *Curr Hypertens Rep* **16:** 499.

Cascella M, Rajnik M, Cuomo A, Dulebohn S C, Di Napoli, R. (2020) Features, Evaluation and Treatment Coronavirus (COVID-19). *StatPearls*. StatPearls Publishing. Available from: https://www.ncbi.nlm.nih.gov/books/NBK554776/

Centers for Disease Control and Prevention. Morbidity and Mortality Weekly Report (mmwr): Preliminary Estimates of the Prevalence of Selected Underlying Health Conditions among Patients with Coronavirus Disease. (accessed on March, 2020), https://www.cdc.gov/mmwr/volumes/69/wr/mm6913e2.htm?s_cid=mm6913e2_w

Chassaing B, Kumar M, Baker M T, Singh V, Vijay-Kumar M (2014) Mammalian gut immunity. *Biomed J* **37(5):** 246–258.

Childs CE, Calder PC, Miles EA (2019) Diet and Immune Function. *Nutrients* **11(8):** 1933.

Corona G, Kreimes A, Barone M *et al.* (2020) Impact of lignans in oilseed mix on gut microbiome composition and enterolignan production in younger healthy and premenopausal women: an in vitro pilot study. *Microb Cell Fact* **19(1):** 82.

Derbyshire E, Delange J (2020) COVID-19: is there a role for immunonutrition, particularly in the over 65s? *BMJ nutr. prev. health* **3(1):** bmjnph-2020-000071.

Devarshi PP, Jangale NM, Ghule AE, Bodhankar SL, Harsulkar AM (2013) Beneficial effects of flaxseed oil and fish oil diet are through modulation of different hepatic genes involved in lipid metabolism in streptozotocin-nicotinamide induced diabetic rats. *Genes Nutr* **8(3):** 329–342.

Dhar D, Mohanty A (2020) Gut microbiota and Covid-19- possible link and implications. *Virus Res* **285:** 198018.

Dzuvor C, Taylor JT, Acquah C, Pan S, Agyei D (2018) Bioprocessing of Functional Ingredients from Flaxseed. *Molecules (Basel, Switzerland)* **23(10):** 2444.

Ejaz H, Alsrhani A, Zafar A, Javed H, Junaid K, Abualgasim E, Khalid OAA, Zeeshan AA, Younas S (2020) COVID-19 and comorbidities: Deleterious impact on infected patients *J Infect Public Health* https://doi.org/10.1016/j.jiph.2020.07.014.

Farrah KM, Farid AS, Mohammed AK (2018) Antioxidant and anti-inflammatory effects of flaxseed oil and fish oil in fipronil induced oxidative stress in rats. *BVMJ* **35(2):** 44-56.

Goyal A, Sharma V, Upadhyay N, Gill S, Sihag M (2014) Flax and flaxseed oil: an ancient medicine & modern functional food. *J Food Sci Technol* **51(9):** 1633–1653.

Granato D, Barba FJ, BursaæKovaèeviæ D, Lorenzo J M, Cruz AG, Putnik P (2020) Functional Foods: Product Development, Technological Trends, Efficacy Testing, and Safety. *Annu Rev Food Sci Technol* **11:** 93–118.

Guan WJ, Liang WH, Zhao Y, Liang HR, Chen ZS, Li YM, Liu XQ, Chen RC, Tang CL, Wang T, Ou CQ, Li L, Chen PY, Sang L, Wang W, Li JF, Li CC, Ou LM, Cheng B, Xiong S (2020) Comorbidity and its impact on 1590 patients with COVID-19 in China: a nationwide analysis. *Eur Respir J* **55(5):** 2000547.

Haghighatsiar N, Askari G, Saraf-Bank S, Feizi A, Keshmiri H (2019) Effect of Flaxseed Powder on Cardiovascular Risk Factor in Dyslipidemic and Hypertensive Patients. *Int J Prev Med* **10:** 218.

Haidari F, Banaei-Jahromi N, Zakerkish M *et al.* (2020) The effects of flaxseed supplementation on metabolic status in women with polycystic ovary syndrome: a randomized open-labeled controlled clinical trial. *Nutr J* **19(8).** 10.1186/s12937-020-0524-5

Hasaniani N, Rahimlou M, RamezaniAhmadi A, MehdizadehKhalifani A, Alizadeh M (2019) The Effect of Flaxseed Enriched Yogurt on the Glycemic Status and Cardiovascular Risk Factors in Patients with Type 2 Diabetes Mellitus: Randomized, Open-labeled, Controlled Study. *ClinNutr Res* **8(4):** 284–295.

He Y, Wang J, Li F, Shi Y (2020) Main Clinical Features of COVID-19 and Potential Prognostic and Therapeutic Value of the Microbiota in SARS-CoV-2 Infections. *Front. Microbiol* **11:** 1302.

Hirayama D, Iida T, Nakase H (2017) The Phagocytic Function of Macrophage-Enforcing Innate Immunity and Tissue Homeostasis. *Int J Mol Sci* **19(1):** 92.

Horowitz R, Freeman PR (2020) Three novel prevention, diagnostic, and treatment options for COVID-19 urgently necessitating controlled randomized trials. *Med Hypotheses* **143:** 109851 - 109851.

Jamilian M, Tabassi Z, Reiner Z, Panahandeh I, Naderi F, Aghadavod E, Amirani E, Taghizadeh M, Shafabakhsh R, Satari M, Mansournia MA, Memarzadeh MR, Asemi Z (2020) The effects of *n*-3 fatty acids from flaxseed oil on genetic and metabolic profiles in patients with gestational diabetes mellitus: a randomised, double-blind, placebo-controlled trial. *Br J Nutr* **123(7):** 792–799.

Kajla P, Sharma A, Sood, DR (2015) Flaxseed-a potential functional food source. *J Food SciTechnol* **52(4):** 1857–1871.

Katare C, Saxena S, Agrawal S, Prasad GBKS, Bisen PS (2012) Flax Seed: A Potential Medicinal Food. *J Nutr Food Sci*, **2:**120.

Khalesi S, Irwin C, Schubert M (2015) Flaxseed consumption may reduce blood pressure: a systematic review and meta-analysis of controlled trials. *J Nutr* **145(4):** 758–765.

Kumar V (2020) Macrophages: The Potent Immunoregulatory Innate Immune Cells. *Intech Open* Doi: 10.5772/intechopen.88013.

Magro G (2020) SARS-CoV-2 and COVID-19: is interleukin-6 (IL-6) the 'culprit lesion' of ARDS onset? What is there besides Tocilizumab? *Cytokine* X2(2): 100029.

Marginã D, Ungurianu A, Purdel C, Nitulescu G M, Tsoukalas D, Sarandi E, Thanasoula M, Burykina TI, Tekos F, Buha A, Nikitovic D, Kouretas D, Tsatsakis AM (2020) Analysis of the intricate effects of polyunsaturated fatty acids and polyphenols on inflammatory pathways in health and disease. *Food Chem Toxicol* **143:** 111558.

Messina G, Polito R, Monda V, Cipolloni L, Di Nunno N, Di Mizio G, Murabito P, Carotenuto M, Messina A, Pisanelli D, Valenzano A, Cibelli G, Scarinci A, Monda M, Sessa F (2020) Functional Role of Dietary Intervention to Improve the Outcome of COVID-19: A Hypothesis of Work. *Int J Mol Sci* **21(9):** 3104.

Mohamed S, Abdelhamid M, Abdel-Aziz M, Montser A (2019) The impact of flaxseed oil active compounds in its native and nano forms on the rat gut microbiota. *Curr Sci Int* DOI: 10.36632/csi/2019.8.4.5.

Mohammadi SM, Mazloom Z, Raeisi-Dehkordi H, BaratiBoldaji R, Bellissimo N, Totosy de ZJ (2017)The effect of flaxseed supplementation on body weight and body composition: A systematic review and meta-analysis of 45 randomized placebo-controlled trials. *Obes Rev* DOI: 10.1111/obr.12550.

Naja F, Hamadeh R (2020) Nutrition amid the COVID-19 pandemic: a multi-level framework for action. *Eur J ClinNutr* **74(8):** 1117–1121.

Ndou SP, Tun HM, Kiarie E *et al.* (2018) Dietary supplementation with flaxseed meal and oat hulls modulates intestinal histomorphometric characteristics, digesta- and mucosa-associated microbiota in pigs. *Sci Rep* **8:** 5880.

Nogueira-de-Almeida CA, Ciampo L, Ferraz IS, Ciampo I, Contini AA, Ued F (2020) COVID-19 and obesity in childhood and adolescence: a clinical review. *J Pediatr (Rio J).* https://doi.org/10.1016/j.jpedp.2020.07.003.

Parikh M, Netticadan T, Pierce GN (2018) Flaxseed: its bioactive components and their cardiovascular benefits. *Am J Physiol Heart CircPhysiol* **314(2):** 146–159.

Ren GY, Chen CY, Chen GC, Chen WG, Pan A, Pan CW, Zhang YH, Qin LQ, Chen LH (2016) Effect of Flaxseed Intervention on Inflammatory Marker C-Reactive Protein: A Systematic Review and Meta-Analysis of Randomized Controlled Trials. *Nutrients* **8(3):** 136.

Rezaei S, Sasani MR, Akhlaghi M, Kohanmoo A (2020) Flaxseed oil in the context of a weight loss programme ameliorates fatty liver grade in patients with non-alcoholic fatty liver disease: a randomised double-blind controlled trial. *Br J Nutr* **123(9):** 994–1002.

Rodriguez-Leyva D, Dupasquier CM, McCullough R, Pierce GN (2010) The cardiovascular effects of flaxseed and its omega-3 fatty acid, alpha-linolenic acid. *Can J Cardiol* **26(9):** 489–496.

Rogero M, Leão M, Santana T, Pimentel M, Carlini G, Silveira T, Gonçalves R, Castro I (2020) Potential benefits and risks of omega-3 fatty acids supplementation to patients with COVID-19. *Free Radic. Biol. Med* DOI: 10.1016/j.freeradbiomed.2020.07.005.

Sanmartin C, Taglieri I, Venturi F., Macaluso, M., Zinnai, A., Tavarini, S., Botto, A., Serra, A., Conte, G., Flamini, G, Angelini LG (2020) Flaxseed Cake as a Tool for the Improvement of Nutraceutical and Sensorial Features of Sourdough Bread. *Foods (Basel, Switzerland)* **9(2):** 204.

Sanyaolu A, Okorie C, Marinkovic A *et al* (2020) Comorbidity and its Impact on Patients with COVID-19. *SN Compr Clin Me* **2:** 1069–1076.

Shakoor H, Feehan J, Al Dhaheri AS, Ali HI, Platat C, Ismail LC, Apostolopoulos V, Stojanovska L (2021) Immune-boosting role of vitamins D, C, E, zinc, selenium and omega-3 fatty acids: Could they help against COVID-19? *Maturitas* **143**: 1–9.

Sherif SM, Mohamed A, Mohamed AA, Ahmed M (2019) The impact of flaxseed oil active compounds in its native and nano forms on the rat gut microbiota. *Curr Sci Int* Doi: 10.36632/csi/2019.8.4.5

Singhal T (2020) A Review of Coronavirus Disease-2019 (COVID-19). *Indian J Pediatr* **87(4)**: 281–286

Szabó, Z, Marosvölgyi T, Szabó É, Bai P, Figler M, Verzár Z (2020) The Potential Beneficial Effect of EPA and DHA Supplementation Managing Cytokine Storm in Coronavirus Disease. *Front Physiol* **11**: 752

Thakur G, Analava M, Kunal P, Derick R (2009) Effect of flaxseed gum on reduction of blood glucose & cholesterol in Type 2 diabetic patients. *Int J Food Sci Nutr* **60**: 1-11.

Ursoniu S, Sahebkar A, Andrica F, Serban C, Banach M, Lipid and Blood Pressure Meta-analysis Collaboration (LBPMC) Group (2016) Effects of flaxseed supplements on blood pressure: A systematic review and meta-analysis of controlled clinical trial. *ClinNutr* **35(3)**: 615–625.

Van der Lelie D, Taghavi S (2020) COVID-19 and the Gut Microbiome: More than a Gut Feeling. *mSystems* **5(4)**. 10.1128/mSystems.00453-20

World Health Organization. COVID-19 significantly impacts health services for noncommunicable diseases. (accessed on 1st June, 2020), https://www.who.int/news-room/detail/01-06-2020-covid-19-significantly-impacts-health-services-for-noncommunicable-diseases

Wu D, Lewis ED, Pae, M, Meydani SN (2019) Nutritional Modulation of Immune Function: Analysis of Evidence, Mechanisms, and Clinical Relevance. *Front Immunol* **9**: 3160.

Yang J, Zheng Y, Gou X, Pu K, Chen, Zhaofeng, Guo Q, Ji R, Wang H, Wang Y, Zhou Y (2020) Prevalence of comorbidities and its effects in patients infected with SARS-CoV-2: a systematic review and meta-analysis. *Int J Infect Dis* **94**: 91-95.

Zarepoor L, Lu JT, Zhang C, Wu W, Lepp D, Robinson L, Wanasundara J, Cui S, Villeneuve S, Fofana B, Tsao R, Wood GA, Power KA (2014) Dietary flaxseed intake exacerbates acute colonic mucosal injury and inflammation induced by dextran sodium sulfate. *Am J Physiol Gastrointest Liver Physiol* **306(12)**: 1042–1055.

Zhang L, Liu Y (2020) Potential interventions for novel coronavirus in China: A systematic review. *J Med Virol* **92(5):** 479–490.

Zhong J, Tang J, Ye C, Dong L (2020) The immunology of COVID-19: is immune modulation an option for treatment? *The Lancet Rheumatology* **2(7):** 428-436.

Zhu L, Sha L, Li K *et al.* (2020) Dietary flaxseed oil rich in omega-3 suppresses severity of type 2 diabetes mellitus via anti-inflammation and modulating gut microbiota in rats. *Lipids Health Dis* https://doi.org/10.1186/s12944-019-1167-4.

Immunity Boosting Functional Foods to Combat COVID-19, Pages: 103–118
Edited by: Apurba Giri
Copyright © 2021, Narendra Publishing House, Delhi, India

C H A P T E R - 9

DRAGON FRUIT: THE NEW FUNCTIONAL FOOD AND ITS POTENTIAL USE IN TREATING CO-MORBID DISEASES IN THE COVID-19 SITUATION

Imana Pal

Ph.D Research Scholar, Department of Home Science, University of Calcutta, Alipore-700027, Kolkata, West Bengal, India
E-mail: imana.pal09@gmail.com

ABSTRACT

COVID-19 is a highly contagious disease and transmitted directly by person to person. There are also several indirect transmissions routes responsible for the transmission of the disease. Though several antiviral drugs such as remdesivir and lopinavir plus ritonavir, and anti-rheumatic drug hydroxychloroquine have been used in clinical practice but their efficacy and safety are still under evaluation. Till now, there is no effective cure for COVID-19 infection; as a result, supportive care is necessary for boosting immunity and prevention of the infection. Studies suggested that functional foods can prevent the mechanism of viral infection as well as act as modulators of immune response. One such food is Dragon fruit, the new super fruit of India. It has gained much popularity due to its eye-catching appearance and nutritive value. They are rich in vitamins, minerals, and antioxidants especially betalains which protect the body from various oxidative stress-related diseases. The polyphenol content of the dragon fruit is also high and the seeds of this fruit are rich in linoleic acid. Studies suggested that dragon fruit had hypocholesterolemic, anti-diabetic, antioxidant, immmuno-boosting, and prebiotic properties which makes the fruit inevitable as a functional food and can be encouraged to consume in this COVID-19 situation as researches indicated that patients suffering from co-morbid diseases have a higher mortality rate if affected with COVID-19 virus. Therefore, the paper tries to investigate how the inclusion of dragon fruit in the diet can improve the body's immunity, reduces the chances of co-morbid diseases, and helps the people fighting in this new normal situation.

Keywords: COVID-19, Antiviral, Antirheumatic, Immune response, Polyphenols, Co-morbid diseases

INTRODUCTION

Novel Coronavirus SARS CoV-2 is responsible for the coronavirus disease or COVID-19. It is an extremely contagious infection that was recognized in December, 2019. WHO declared the infection as pandemic on 11th March, 2020 (WHO, 2020). Over 9, 25,301 deaths and over 2.8 million corresponding cases of COVID-19 have been recorded in more than 215 nations and the numbers of infected cases are growing at a rapid rate (Worldometer, 2020). Since COVID-19 is a new disease and researches are still going on, the data available on the disease is inadequate. However, observations of several cases indicated that underlying co-morbid diseases increase the possibility of this viral infection. Currently available information and clinical expertise showed that aged people particularly those who are hospitalized for a long time and individuals of any age group having underlying serious health conditions are susceptible to coronavirus infection. It has also been seen that both the infection rate and death rate are high in the elderly population as well as people having chronic medical conditions such as hyperglycaemia, heart, or lung diseases (BCCDC, 2020). People suffering from uncontrolled health conditions like hypertension, hyperglycaemia, pulmonary, hepatic, and kidney diseases, cancer patients receiving chemotherapy, patients with organ transplantation, and patients who are on steroids are at a higher risk of having COVID-19 infection.

Till date, no successful cure for COVID-19 has been invented, so the scientists and authorities are trying to seek information and searching for the present and long term cure of the current and upcoming pandemic fiasco individually.

Food is a basic necessity for human survival and cannot be locked down, so food sectors and its stakeholders are also in the limelight (Huff *et al.*, 2015). Lack of appropriate treatment also make the consumers think about adopting a healthier diet rich in immuno-boosting foods and functional foods whose bioactive ingredients are believed to enhance the immune function, gives protection against co-morbid diseases such as diabetes mellitus, hypertension, cardiovascular diseases, cancer, other oxidative stress related diseases and help fight off viruses, as a result, the demands for these foods are increasing (Naik *et al.*, 2010; Gibson *et al.*, 2012). Consumption of fresh vegetables and fruits rich in vitamins and minerals, antioxidants, and functional foods are of immense importance in this context. For example, Vitamin C (Ascorbic acid) plays a protective role by supporting the immune function of the body as well as necessary for repairing the wear and tear of body tissues (Carr *et al.*, 2017). It also helps to inhibit the lower respiratory tract infection under certain conditions (Hemilä *et al.*, 1997). Vitamin A, another important vitamin, is a mixture of fat-soluble compounds (including beta carotene, retinol, and retinoic acid) that helps the body to fight against infection and boost immune function (Huang *et al.*, 2018). It has also been seen that Vitamin D and Vitamin E supplementation may counteract the COVID-19 infection (Wang *et al.*, 2020). Dietary supplementation with these vitamins, minerals, and other bioactive compounds may assist the immune system of the human body to fight against COVID-19 (Consumer Research Supports, 2020).

Enormous investigation and improvement measures were able to invent a large number of synthetic molecules useful for medicinal purposes. Yet the detrimental consequences of those emerge as a huge difficulty which causes a shift in the utilization of herbal products. The application of bioactive elements of natural sources especially plants have been used from prehistoric times. Herbal products have been used as first-line therapy, supplements, or curative support alongside allopathic medicine. Researches on natural medicines have gained much attention in recent times (Salehi *et al.*, 2018; Sharifi –Rad *et al.*, 2018a, b; Salehi *et al.*, 2019). Dragon fruit is one of those fruits that have been catching attention in recent decades. Dragon fruits are known to have both nutraceutical and therapeutic properties. Natural products containing bioactive phytochemicals that can be used for the formulation of a nutraceutical is called functional foods and dragon fruit have all the properties, therefore it is considered as functional food.

At present, 'Dragon fruit' or 'Pitaya' becomes popular because of their health promoting activities and economic potential. The fruit is called "Buah-Naga" in Malay and belongs to the Cactaceae family and genus Hylocereus (Bellec *et al.*, 2006; Jaafar *et al.*, 2009; Nurul *et al.*, 2014). The fruit is oval shaped and its outer peel has a scaly appearance (Wybraniec, 2001; Nurul *et al.*, 2014). The fresh dragon fruits are sweet and juicy with many small comestible black coloured seeds.

Commercially, three types of dragon fruit are cultivated (Lim *et al.*, 2012; Nurul *et al.*, 2014). The differentiation is done according to their size, shape, and colour of the flesh (Bellec *et al.*, 2006). The most common is red pitaya or *Hylocereus polyrhizus,* as the name depicts it contains both red peel and flesh with lots of edible and soft seeds (Stintzing *et al.*, 2002). *H. undatus* or white pitaya has white flesh (Bellec *et al.*, 2006; Lim *et al.*, 2012). The third type is *H. megalanthus*, also called the yellow pitaya consisting of white flesh and yellow skin (Bellec *et al.*, 2006; Lim *et al.*, 2012). Researches indicated that hybridization of *Hylocereus costaricensis* and *Selenicerus inermis* produced yellow pitaya (Tel-zur *et al.*, 2004) which is medicinally less valuable compared to the other two varieties. But the edible seeds of yellow dragon fruit are rich in PUFA (Chemah *et al.*, 2010). Yellow dragon fruit is indigenous to Colombia and Peru and seldom transported to Europe and Canada (Lim *et al.*, 2012). Red dragon fruit is supposed to be originated in Costa Rica (Bellec *et al.*, 2006, Lim *et al.*, 2012) and nowadays it is mostly cultivated in South East Asia (Rebecca *et al.*, 2010) for its health and economic benefits. *H. polyrhizus* exerts its health promoting effects as it is rich in vitamins (Bellec *et al.*, 2006; Jaafar *et al.*, 2009; Lim *et al.*, 2012) and minerals (Jaafar *et al.*, 2009; Khalili *et al.*, 2009) as well as in red betacyanin, a nitrogen containing compound, which is present in its peel and flesh (Vaillant *et al.*, 2005; Rebecca *et al.*, 2010; Angaji, 2012; Lim *et al.*, 2012; Tenore *et al.*, 2012) Betacyanin has antioxidant properties and very much effective against diseases linked with oxidative stress (Rebecca *et al.*, 2010; Lim *et al.*, 2012; Liaotrakoon *et al.*, 2013; Nurul *et al.*, 2014). In addition to this, red dragon fruit also contains linoleic acid, an essential fatty acid with numerous physiological benefits (Khalili *et al.*, 2009; Lim *et al.*, 2012). On the other hand, the white dragon fruit is generally larger than the red one and is thought to be originated in the southern part of Mexico and now its cultivation has spread across Asian nations such as Malaysia, Taiwan, Vietnam as well as northern Australia. The nutritional composition of white pitaya is almost similar to the red pitaya except it contains a greater amount of moisture, protein, fats, and fibre. *H.undatus* is also rich in antioxidants which make it significant to health (Lim *et al.*, 2012).

Free Radicals, Oxidative Stress and their Roles in Co-morbid Diseases

Free radicals on oxidative stress

Free radicals are substances produced from compounds that are partially oxidized and that have undergone incomplete burning. Free radicals have oxygen groups in their structure which can start oxidation reactions both at the cell membrane surface and inside the cells. Free radicals are produced in the body either from endogenous processes (incomplete catabolism, production of energy, detoxification of the liver, etc.) or from exogenous sources (smoke of a cigarette, air pollution, foods, drugs, or water, etc.). Free radicals have unpaired electrons which make them unstable and reactive because they want to stabilize themselves by pairing with electrons taken from other compounds. They interact with the macromolecules causing cell damage and homeostatic imbalance (Butnariu *et al.*, 2012).

Oxidative stress can be defined as a state of oxidative injury resulting from inequality between the generation of free radical and antioxidant resistance. Oxidative stress is currently thought to make a significant contribution to co-morbid diseases (Lobo et al., 2010) which inturn worsens the health condition of COVID-19 patients.

Effect on diabetes

Oxidative stress is a crucial reason in producing a large range of medical conditions such as cancer, heart diseases, hyperglycaemia, aging, hepatic, and respiratory tract diseases. The main reason behind oxidative stress is the inequality between radical producing and radical scavenging activities. Defect in the free radical generation and faulty antioxidant protection mechanism are the two main reasons behind diabetes mellitus (Opara et al., 2002). Pro-oxidant, antioxidant imbalance which is the main reason behind the pathogenesis of diabetes occurs due to the auto-oxidation of glucose, excess production of glycation end products (AGEs), the pathway of polyol, hexamine, and mitochondrial respiratory chain. The enzymatic sources of free radical production are nitric oxide synthase, xanthine oxidase, and NADPH oxidase (Singh et al., 2009).

Effect on cancer

The causation of cancer in individual is a complex process involving a combination of endogenous and exogenous factors that mediate molecular and cell changes. Oxidative DNA damage has been proven to be responsible for the development of cancer (Valko et al., 2004; Valko et al., 2006; Valko et al., 2007). Initiation and promotion of cancer are linked to chromosomal defects and free radical-induced activation of oncogenes. A significant event in chemical carcinogenesis is the production of hydroxyled bases of DNA (Valko et al., 2004; Halliwell, 2007) as a common type of damage. The induction of genetic mutation and modification of normal gene transcription causes disturbance in the growth of normal cells. Several alterations in the structure of DNA, including base and sugar lesions, breakage of the strand, cross-linking of DNA protein and base-free sites, are also caused by oxidative DNA injury. For instance, chronic cigarette smoking and inflammation caused by non-infectious diseases, such as asbestos, can cause oxidative DNA injury that can lead to lung cancer and other tumour development (Valko et al., 2004; Willcox et al., 2004). The important link between fat and leukaemia, breast, ovary, and rectum cancers death rates in seniors may indicate increased lipid peroxidation (Young et al., 2001; Droge, 2002).

Effect on cardiovascular diseases

There are several reasons for the occurrence of cardiovascular diseases and a variety of risk factors are responsible for the causation of the diseases. The major risk factors include high blood pressure, hypercholesterolemia, hyperglycaemia, smoking, unhealthy diet, mental stress, and lack of physical activity (Droge, 2002; Bahorun *et al.*, 2006; Ceriello, 2008). Recently, researches raised a controversy about whether the role of oxidative stress is considered as a primary or secondary reason for several cardiovascular complications (Ceriello, 2008). Further in vivo and in vitro experiments gave useful support and proved that oxidative stress was a key factor for various CVDs namely hypertension, atherosclerosis, cardiomyopathy, cardiac hypertrophy, ischemia, and congestive cardiac failure (Droge, 2002; Bahorun *et al.*, 2006; Chatterjee *et al.*, 2007; Ceriello, 2008)

Effect on pulmonary disease

Inflammatory lung disorders like asthma and Chronic Obstructive Pulmonary Disease (COPD) are characterized by systemic and local chronic inflammation and oxidative stress (MacNee, 2001; Caramori *et al.*, 2004; Guo *et al.*, 2007; Hoshino *et al.*, 2008). Oxidants can enhance inflammation by activating specific kinases and redox transcription factors such as NF-kappa B and AP-1 (MacNee, 2001; Hoshino *et al.*, 2008)

Effect on renal diseases

One of the most important reasons for multiple kidney disorders such as glomerulonephritis and tubule-interstitial nephritis, chronic kidney failure, proteinuria, uremia is oxidative stress. Nephrotoxic effects of various medicines like cyclosporine, tacrolimus (FK506), gentamycin, bleomycin, vinblastine, is primarily because of oxidative stress caused by lipid peroxidation. Various types of heavy metals (Pb, Cd, As, Hg) and transition metals (Cu, Fe, Cr, Co) produce diverse types of nephropathy and carcinogenic reactions by inducing free radicals in the body (Pham-Huy *et al.*, 2008).

Dragon Fruit-Phytochemical Composition and Health Benefits

The presence of a large quantity of polyphenolic compounds and antioxidant activity make dragon fruit popular among cultivars worldwide (Hor *et al.*, 2012). Polyphenolic compounds provide antioxidant activity and perform as bioactive scavengers of free radicals, thus playing an important function in the protection of the human body (Barros *et al.*, 2015). Antioxidants can be defined as compounds having the ability to inhibit oxidation of proteins, lipids, and nucleic acid molecules by interrupting the initiation of oxidative chain reaction and its propagation, thereby defending the body cells from the harmful effects of oxidative injury (Sumino *et al.*, 2002; Valentão *et al.*, 2002). Two most important fruit pigments, red-violet coloured betacyanins, or yellow coloured betaxanthines, belonging to betalain pigments are present in Dragon fruit (Stintzing *et al.*, 2002). Betalains are a group of chemical compounds. They have both antioxidant properties and radical scavenging activities (Wong *et al.*, 2015).

Another important antioxidant present in Dragon fruit is ascorbic acid or vitamin C. It is involved in several physiological activities in living organisms, such as it acts as a reducing agent and prevents the oxidative damage in cellular components (Karamac *et al.*, 2006). This is because ascorbic acid can oxidize free radicals and oxygen-derived cells as scavengers like H_2O_2, singlet oxygen, and hydroxyl radicals (Duarte *et al.*, 2005). Hence, ascorbic acid is used in the management of photo-aging (Vaiserman, 2008). Rather, ascorbic acid's pro-oxidant properties also support its antibacterial activity (Villacorta *et al.*, 2007).

Exogenous stimulation and regulation of various enzymes augmented the creation of both free radicals as well as antioxidants in the human body. If free radicals are extensively formed, trauma, inflammation, and other chronic ailments like cancer, and degenerative diseases can occur as a result of oxidative stress (Aguirre *et al.*, 2008). In recent decades, a few antioxidant vitamins have been introduced that can limit oxidative damage, such as β-carotene, vitamin C, and vitamin E (Gey *et al.*, 1993). It was observed in various epidemiological studies that there exists a close relationship between low beta carotene level, tocopherol, and ascorbic acid level in plasma and heart disease (Hajer *et al.*, 2007). This can be seen in epidemiological studies by the strong association between heart disease and low plasma levels of β-carotene, tocopherol, and l-ascorbic acid.

Several studies documented the health benefits of various parts of dragon fruit, viz. flesh, seeds, and peel. This analysis, therefore, summarises some health benefits of dragon fruit such as antioxidant, anticancer, glucose, and cholesterol lowering properties and prebiotic effect which reduce the chances of co-morbidity.

Antioxidant property

The body's vital molecules such as DNA are damaged by reactive oxygen species (ROS) namely, hydrogen peroxide, hydroxyl radicals, superoxide anions which leads to the death of the cells and injury to the tissues. Consequently, antioxidants such as polyphenols, tocopherols, and flavonoids play a crucial role in retarding or hindering oxidation of cellular components. Free radical scavenging activity of a food is directly proportional to the high total phenolic content (TPC). Previous researches revealed that the chief antioxidant compounds present in Hylocerus sp. are polyphenols. These compounds act as reducing agents and ended the chain reaction by donating electrons to the free radicals. In addition to that, their antioxidant properties have been attributed to their singlet oxygen quencher effects and metal chelating properties. Moreover, betacyanin and flavonoids like kaempferol, quercetin, and isorhamnetin present in the flesh of dragon fruit show radical scavenging and metal chelating abilities.

Generally, the antioxidant properties of pitaya peel were superior compared to its flesh because of the difference of bioactive ingredients of pitaya peel and flesh. The peel mostly contains flavonoids whereas the flesh is rich in non-flavonoid compounds and this difference is responsible for the disparity of antioxidant activities of different parts of the fruit. The total phenolic content of red dragon fruit was higher compared to the white one because red flesh is rich in phenolic compounds and betalains and has higher antioxidant activities.

In short, Hylocereus species show potential antioxidant activities that provide health benefits (Choo *et al.*, 2016).

Hypocholesterolemic properties

The cholesterol-lowering property of dragon fruit is due to its polyphenols content. Interaction between free radicals and lipids inside the body produces lipid peroxidase which causes oxidation of LDL. This oxidized LDL reacts with platelets and causes the production of foam cells which in turn increases the chance of atherosclerosis. Polyphenols present in the dragon fruit were found to prevent lipid peroxidation and oxidation of LDL and reduced the risk of cardiac diseases. Polyphenols also reduce the chance of clotting of blood which also aids in the prevention of heart diseases. Several animal experiments indicated that dragon fruit exhibited cardioprotective properties because of its antioxidant content (Choo *et al.*, 2016).

The nutritional analysis showed that dragon fruit contains a small amount of cholesterol, saturated fat and, trans fat. Therefore, the consumption of this fruit helps to maintain a healthy heart. Seeds of dragon fruits are rich in þ-3 and þ-6 fatty acids and PUFAs which also exert health benefits. The combined effect of the above factors makes the dragon fruit a good choice (Sinha *et al.*, 2018).

Immunity boosting properties

Dragon fruit is a rich source of ascorbic acid, B vitamins, flavonoids, and minerals like phosphorus, calcium, iron, and other bioactive compounds that act as antioxidants that have free radical scavenging properties and help to maintain a strong immune function of the body. The flesh and peel extract of dragon fruits (both red and white) are the source of proteins and polyphenols which makes it an immune-boosting food and indispensable as functional food and nutraceutical. Dragon fruits also can restore and enhance the number of WBC in the body that protects the body from toxins and prevent the growth of pathogenic microorganisms. Therefore, improvement of wound healing and immuno-boosting ability of the body can be enhanced by the consumption of dragon fruit (Sinha *et al.*, 2018).

Anticancer activity

Research evidence indicated the presence of flavonoids, polyphenols, and betalains are responsible for cancer preventing properties of Hylocereus species, though the exact mechanism of cancer preventing mechanism is still remains unidentified. However, it is believed that cancer preventing properties of dragon fruit can be mediated through suppression of nuclear factor kB and growth factor receptor mediated pathway; arrest of cell cycle and induction of apoptosis; inhibition of angiogenesis and mitogen activated protein kinase; as well as antioxidant and anti-inflammatory mechanism (Choo *et al.*, 2016).

Prebiotic effect

Prebiotic can be defined as the oligosaccharides that are non-digestible and stimulate the multiplication of colon flora which inturn beneficial for the health of the host. Several studies revealed that the use of prebiotics can give protection against colon cancer and decreases the tendency of inflammatory bowel diseases. Growth of lactobacilli and bifidobacteria, the most important gut micro flora can prevent the growth of pathogenic microorganisms in the gastrointestinal tract and maintains the health of the digestive tract (Choo *et al.*, 2016).

Hypoglycaemic effect

Diabetes mellitus is a metabolic disorder responsible for a large number of deaths around the world. Researches are going on the use of natural and herbal medicines in the treatment of diabetes and the sector is booming. White dragon fruit has an inhibitory effect of cAMP phosphorylase that inturn retains insulin for a long period. Phytoconstituents present in dragon fruit can effectively lower blood sugar levels. The flavonoid content of dragon fruit is responsible for its glucose lowering property which is mediated by three mechanisms, namely, reduction of oxidative stress by its antioxidant activity, suppression of GLUT2 in intestinal mucosa and phosphodiesterase thereby augmented retention of insulin. Studies conducted by researchers proved that regular intake of red pitaya or red dragon fruit effectively controls blood sugar level and keeps the lipid profile level under control in patients suffering from Type II diabetes or NIDDM. Type II diabetes is often connected with obesity as it causes insulin resistance. White dragon fruit juice is effective in controlling insulin resistance, a metabolic disorder associated with obesity. It was also found that aqueous extract of *H. undatus* reduced the complications related to diabetes. Thus, it can be said that dragon fruit can not only be used in the prevention and treatment of hyperglycaemia but also effective in controlling its complications (Joshi *et al.*, 2020)

Nutraceutical activity

A nutraceutical can be defined as a combination of the food and pharmaceutical industries. These are functional foods that provide nutrients along with added health benefits. Nutraceuticals include pre and probiotics, dietary fibre, antioxidants, polyphenols, vitamins, polyunsaturated fatty acids, and spices (Das *et al.*, 2012). Dragon fruit's nutraceutical property can be attributed to its vitamins, antioxidants, polyphenols, PUFA, and prebiotic properties. Dragon fruit is an excellent source of protein, fat, antioxidants, and dietary fibre. Whole dragon fruit is used for the preparation of dragon fruit powder that can be used as a health supplement (Tze *et al.*, 2012).

CONCLUSION

Pitaya or dragon fruit is enriched with phytoconstituents. Every part of the fruit i.e. peels, flesh and seeds have pharmacological benefits and nutraceutical properties. Therapeutic benefits of dragon fruit include antioxidant, anticancer, hypoglycemic, and cardioprotective properties which protect the body from co-morbid diseases that makes people susceptible to COVID-19 infection. Besides these, the fruit also exhibits prebiotic effects, demonstrating the fruit's nutraceutical benefits. The fruit can be used as a natural colourant in edible food products because of its high betacyanin content. Thus, dragon fruit can be considered as a super fruit and focused investigation on this wonder fruit is expected to better control many new age life-threatening diseases including COVID-19.

REFERENCES

Aguirre R, May JM (2008) Inflammation in the vascular bed: importance of vitamin C. *Pharmacol Therap* **119(1)**: 96-103.

Angaji SA (2012) Antioxidants: a few key points. *Ann Biol Res* **3(8)**: 3968-77.

Bahorun T, Soobrattee MA, Luximon-Ramma V, Aruoma OI (2006) Free radicals and antioxidants in cardiovascular health and disease. *Int J Med Update* **1(2)**: 25-41

Barros A, Gironés-Vilaplana A, Texeira A, Baenas N, Domínguez-Perles R (2015) Grape stems as a source of bioactive compounds: application towards added-value commodities and significance for human health. *Phytochem Rev* **14(6)**: 921-931.

BCCDC (2020). COVID-19 vulnerable populations. British Columbia Centre for Disease Control. Web. http://www.bccdc.ca/health-info/diseases-conditions/covid-19/vulnerable-populations (accessed 18th April, 2020).

Bellec FL, Vaillant F, Imbert E (2006) Pitahaya (Hylocereus spp.): a new fruit crop, a market with a future. *Fruits* **61(4)**: 237-250.

Butnariu M, Samfira I (2012) Free radicals and oxidative stress. *J Bioequiv Availab* **4(6)**: 4-6.

Caramori G, Papi A (2004) Oxidants and asthma. *Thorax* **59(2)**: 170-173

Carr AC, Maggini S (2017) Vitamin C and immune function. *Nutr* **9(11)**: 1211.

Centers for Disease Control and Prevention (2020) Coronavirus (COVID-19): symptoms of coronavirus Web. https://www.cdc.gov/coronavirus/2019-ncov/symptoms-testing/symptoms.html (accessed 18th April, 2020).

Ceriello A (2008) Possible role of oxidative stress in the pathogenesis of hypertension. *Diabetes Care* **31 (Suppl 2)**: S181-184.

Chatterjee M, Saluja R, Kanneganti S, Chinta S, Dikshit M (2007). Biochemical and molecular evaluation of neutrophil NOS in spontaneously hypertensive rats. *Cell Mol biol* **53(1)**: 84-93.

Chemah TC, Aminah A, Noriham A, Wan Aida WM (2010) Determination of pitaya seeds as a natural antioxidant and source of essential fatty acids. *Int Food Res J* **17**: 1003-1010.

Choo JC, Koh RY, Ling APK (2016). Medicinal properties of pitaya: a review. *Spatula DD* **6(2)**: 69-76.

Consumer Research Supports Global Demand for Immunity Products Web. https://www.naturalproductsinsider.com/business-resources/consumer-research-supports-globaldemand-immunity-products-white-paper (accessed on 13th April 2020).

Countries where Coronavirus has Spread—Worldometer Web. https://www.worldo meters.info/coronavirus/countries-where-coronavirus-has-spread/ (accessed on 13th September 2020).

Das L, Bhaumik E, Raychaudhuri U, Chakraborty R (2012) Role of nutraceuticals in human health. *J Food Sci Technol* **49(2):** 173–183.

Droge W (2002) Free radicals in the physiological control of cell function. *Physiol Rev* **82(1):** 47-95.

Duarte TL, Lunec J (2005). When is an antioxidant not an antioxidant? A review of novel actions and reactions of vitamin C. *Free Rad Res* **39(7):** 671-686.

Gey KF, Moser UK, Jordan P, Stähelin HB, Eichholzer M, Lüdin E (1993). Increased risk of cardiovascular disease at suboptimal plasma concentrations of essential antioxidants: an epidemiological update with special attention to carotene and vitamin C. *Am J Clin Nutr* **57(5):** 787S-797S.

Gibson A, Edgar JD, Neville CE, Gilchrist SECM, McKinley MC, Patterson CC, Young IS, Woodside JV (2012) Effect of fruit and vegetable consumption on immune function in older people: A randomized controlled trial. *Am J Clin Nutr* **96**: 1429–1436.

Guo RF, Ward PA (2007) Role of oxidants in lung injury during sepsis. *Antioxid Redox Signal* **9(11):** 1991-2002.

Hajer GR, van der Graaf Y, Olijhoek JK, Edlinger M, Visseren FL (2007) Low plasma levels of adiponectin are associated with low risk for future cardiovascular events in patients with clinical evident vascular disease. *Am Heart J* **154(4):** 750-e1-750-e7.

Hemilä H (1997) Vitamin C intake and susceptibility to pneumonia. *Pediatr Infect Dis J* **16**: 836–837.

Hor SY, Ahmed M, Farsi E, Yam MF, Hashim MA (2012) Safety Assessment of Methanol Extract of Red Dragon Fruit (Hylocereus polyrhizus): Acute and Subchronic Toxicity Studies. *Regulatory Toxicol and Pharmacol* **63(1):** 106-114.

Hoshino Y, Mishima M (2008) Antioxidants & redox signaling redox-based therapeutics for lung diseases. *Antioxid Redox Signal* **10(4):** 701- 704.

Huang Z, Liu Y, Qi G, Brand D, Zheng S (2018) Role of Vitamin A in the Immune System. *J Clin Med* **7(9)**: 258.

Huff AG, Beyeler WE, Kelley NS, McNitt JA (2015) How resilient is the United States' food system to pandemics? *J Environ Stud Sci* **5**: 337–347.

Jaafar RA, Abdul Rahman AR, Che Mahmood NZ, Vasudevan R (2009) Proximate analysis of dragon fruit (Hylecereus polyrhizus). *Am J Applied Sci* **6(7):** 1341-1346.

Joshi M, Prabhakar B (2020) Phytoconstituents and pharmaco therapeutic benefits of pitaya: A wonder fruit. *J Food Biochem* https://doi.org/10.1111/jfbc.13260.

Karamac M, Kosiñska A, Pegg RB (2006) Content of gallic acid in selected plant extracts. *Polish J Food Nutri Sci* **15(1)**: 55.

Khalili MA, Norhayati AH, Rokiah MY, Asmah R, Siti Muskinah M, Abdul Manaf A (2009) Hypocholestrolemia effects of red pitaya (*Hylocereus* sp.) on hypercholestrolemic- induced rat. *Int Food Res J* **16(3)**: 431-440.

Liaotrakoon W, Clereq ND, Hoed VV, Walle DV, Lewille B, Dewettinck K (2013) Impact of thermal treatment on physiochemical, antioxidant and rheological properties of white- flesh and red flesh dragon fruit (*Hylocereus* spp.) purees. *Food Bioprocess Technol* **6(2)**: 416-430.

Lim TK (2012) Edible medicinal and nonmedicinal plants. **In**: H. polyrhizus. 1st edition, Springer, Dordrecht, pp 640-55.

Lobo V, Patil A, Phatak A, Chandra N (2010) Free radicals, antioxidants and functional foods: Impact on human health. *Phcog Rev* **4(8)**: 118.

MacNee W (2001) Oxidative stress and lung inflammation in airways disease. *Eur J Pharmacol* **429(1-3)**: 195-207.

Naik SR, Thakare VN, Joshi FP (2010) Functional foods and herbs as potential immune adjuvants and medicines in maintaining healthy immune system: A commentary. *J Complement Integr Med* **7(1)** https://doi.org/10.2202/1553-3840.1441

Nurul SR, Asmah R (2014) Variability in nutritional composition and phytochemicals properties of red pitaya (Hylocereus polyrhizus) from Malaysia and Australia. *Int Food Res J* **21(4)**: 1689-1697.

Opara EC (20020 Oxidative stress, micronutrients, diabetes mellitus and its complications. *J R Soc Promot Health* **122(1)**:28-34.

Pham-Huy LA, He H, Pham-Huy C (2008). Free radicals, antioxidants in disease and health. *Int J Biomed Sci* **4(2)**: 89.

Prabhakar PK, Doble M (2008) A target based therapeutic approach towards diabetes mellitus using medicinal plants. *Curr Diabet Rev* **4(4)**: 291-308.

Rebecca OPS, Boyce AN, Chandran S (2010) Pigment identification and antioxidant properties of red dragon fruit. *Afr J Biotechnol* **9(10)**: 1450-1454.

Salehi B, Fokou PVT, Sharifi-Rad M, Zucca P, Pezzani R, Martins N, Sharifi-Rad J (2019) The therapeutic potential of naringenin: A review of clinical trials. *Pharmaceuticals* **12(1)**: 11.

Salehi B, Sharopov F, Martorell M, Rajkovic J, Ademiluyi AO, Sharifi-Rad M, Sharifi-Rad J (2018) Phytochemicals in Helicobacter pylori infections: What are we doing now? *Int J Mol Sci* **19(8)**: 2361.

Sharifi-Rad M, Roberts TH, Matthews KR, Bezerra, CF, Morais- Braga MFB, Coutinho HDM, Sharifi-Rad J (2018a) Ethnobotany of the genus Taraxacum— Phytochemicals and antimicrobial activity. *Phytother Res* **32(11)**: 2131–2145.

Sharifi-Rad J, Sharifi-Rad M, Salehi B, Iriti M, Roointan A, Mnayer D, Afshari A (2018b) In vitro and in vivo assessment of free radical scavenging and antioxidant activities of Veronica persica Poir. *Cell Mol Biol* **64(8)**: 57–64.

Singh PP, Mahadi F, Roy A, Sharma P (2009) Reactive nitrogen species and antioxidants in etiopathogenesis of diabetes mellitus Type 2. *Indian J Clin Biochem* **24(4)**:324-342.

Sinha R, Jha MK, Karuna K (2018) Dragon Fruit: A fruit for health benefits and nutritional security. *Int J Agric Sci Res* **8(2)**: 97-100.

Stintzing FC, Schieber A, Carle R (2002) Betacyanins in fruits from red-purple pitaya, Hylocereus polyrhizus (Weber) Britton & Rose. *Food Chem* **77(1)**: 101-106.

Sumino M, Sekine T, Ruangrungsi N, Igarashi K, Ikegami F (2002) Ardisiphenols and other antioxidant principles from the fruits of Ardisia colorata. *Chem Pharm Bull* **50(11)**: 1484-1487.

Tel-zur N, Abbo S, Barozvi D, Mizrahi Y (2004) Genetic relationship among Hylocereus and Selenicereus vine cacti (Cacracear): evidence from hybridisation and cytological studies. *Ann Bot* **94(4)**: 527-534.

Tenore GC, Novellino E, Basile A (2012) Nutraceutical potential and antioxidant benefits of red pitaya (Hylocereus polyrhizus) extracts. *J Funct Foods* **4(1)**: 129-136.

Tze NL, Han CP, Yusof YA, Ling CN, Talib RA, Taip FS, Aziz MG (2012) Physicochemical and nutritional properties of spray-dried pitaya fruit powder as natural colorant. *Food Sci Biotechnol* **21(3)**: 675–682.

Vaillant F, Perez A, Davila I, Dornier M, Reynes M (2005) Colorant and antioxidant properties of red-purple pitahaya. *Fruits* **60(1)**: 3-12.

Vaiserman AM (2008) Life extension by anti-aging drugs: hormetic explanation. *Am J Pharmacol Toxicol* **3**: 14-18.

Valentão P, Fernandes E, Carvalho F, Andrade PB, Seabra RM, Bastos ML (2002) Antioxidative properties of cardoon (Cynara cardunculus L.) infusion against superoxide radical, hydroxyl radical, and hypochlorous acid. *J Agri Food Chem* **50(17)**: 4989-4993.

Valko M, Izakovic M , Mazur M, Rhodes CJ, Telser J (2004) Role of oxygen radicals in DNA damage and cancer incidence. *Mol Cell Biochem* **266 (1-2)**: 37-56.

Valko M, Leibfritz D, Moncol J, Cronin MT, Mazur M, Telser J (2007) Free radicals and antioxidants in normal physiological functions and human disease. *Int J Biochem Cell Biol* **39(1)**: 44-84.

Valko M, Rhodes C, Moncol J, Izakovic MM, Mazur M (2006). Free radicals, metals and antioxidants in oxidative stress-induced cancer. *Chem Biol Interact* **160(1)**: 1-40.

Villacorta L, Azzi A, Zingg JM (2007) Regulatory role of vitamins E and C on extracellular matrix components of the vascular system. *Mol Aspects Med* **28(5-6)**: 507-537.

Wang L,Wang Y, Ye D, Liu Q (2020) A review of the 2019 Novel Coronavirus (COVID-19) based on current evidence. *Int J Antimicrob Agents* https:/ /doi.org/10.1016/j.ijantimicag.2020.105948

Willcox JK, Ash SL, Catignani GL (2004) Antioxidants and prevention of chronic disease. *Crit Rev Food Sci Nutr* **44(4)**: 275-295.

WHO Director-General's Opening Remarks at the Media Briefing on COVID-19—11 March (2020) Web. https://www.who.int/dg/speeches/detail/who-director-general-s- opening-remarks-at-the-mediabriefing-on-covid-19—11-march-2020 (accessed on 13th April 2020).

Wong YM, Siow LF (2015) Effects of heat, pH, antioxidant, agitation and light on betacyanin stability using red-fleshed dragon fruit (Hylocereus polyrhizus) juice and concentrate as models. *J Food Sci Technol* **52(5)**: 3086-3092.

Wybraniec S, Platzner I, Geresh S, Gottlieb HE, Haimberg M, Mogilnitzki M, Mizrahi Y (2001). Betacyanins from vine cactus Hylocereus polyrhizus. *Phytochem* **58(8)**: 1209-1212.

Yeh GY, Eisenberg DM, Kaptchuk TJ, Phillips RS (2003) Systematic review of herbs and dietary supplements for glycemic control in diabetes. *Diabetes Care* **26(4)**: 1277- 1294.

Young I, Woodside J (2001) Antioxidants in health and disease. *J Clin Pathol* **54(3)**: 176- 186.

Immunity Boosting Functional Foods to Combat COVID-19, Pages: 119–132
Edited by: Apurba Giri

CHAPTER - 10

MUSHROOM EXOPOLYSACCHARIDES: THEIR ANTIOXIDANT AND ANTIVIRAL PROPERTIES TO BOOST IMMUNITY AGAINST COVID-19

Trupti K Vyas[1]*, Priya Vadnerker[2], Ridhhi Bhavsar[3] and Kruti Kheni[4]

[1]*Assistant Professor, Food Quality Testing Laboratory,*
Navsari Agricultural University, Navsari-396450, Gujarat, India
E-mail: vyastrupti@hotmail.com
[2]*Microbiologist, Elite Pharma Pvt. Ltd., Ahmedabad-382445, Gujarat, India*
[3]*M. Sc. student (Ex), P D Patel Institute of Applied Sciences,*
CHARUSAT, Changa-388001, Gujarat, India
[4]*Microbiologist, SCHAMKA Technology Ltd, Vadodara-380054, Gujarat, India*
*Corresponding author

ABSTRACT

Medicinal mushrooms are widely used since ancient time to treat many diseases. More than 2500 species of edible or medicinal mushroom are identified and many consumed in culinary items. Many mushroom produced inctracellular polysaccharide (ICP) and exopolysaccharide (EPS) molecules which has immunomodulating properties. This polysaccharide can be homopolymer or heteropolymer and are categorized as glycoprotein or proteoglycans. These polysaccharides contain glucans linked by β-(1-3), (1-6) glycosidic bonds and α-(1-3) glycosidic and these β-glucans have antiviral and anticancer activities. Diverse mushroom produce unique EPS and according to structural dynamics they offer health benefits. These bioactive polysaccharides have potential to fight with cancer, virus, pathogens and have an immune-modulatory effect. EPS posses strong antioxidant activities and thus prevent damage from reactive oxygen species and increase immunity of cell. EPS is well characterized for their health benefits from various edible and medicinal mushroom like *Pleurotus, Trametes, Morchella, Ganoderma, Agaricus, Cordyceps, Lentinus, Grifola* etc., are reported. Moreover, some lectin produced by mushroom which binds with sugar present in carbohydrate are reported for their antiviral activity against plant and human virus like TMV, HIV, Hepatitis A Virus. Hence these fungal EPS are subject of interest in the field of science and industry. In present COVID-19 pandemic consumption of mushroom may be good option to boost immunomodulatory effect.

Keywords: Antioxidant, Antiviral, COVID-19, Exopolysaccharide, Mushrooms

INTRODUCTION

Mushrooms, a fruiting body of fungi, are mostly seen in monsoon season which contain a cap and a stem. On the lower side of the fruiting body it contains gill having spore to spread in nature. Mushroom can be classified into several categories as per their different uses. These fruiting bodies containing mushroom can be classified based on their use classified in major three categories, i.e., medicinal, edible and poisonous mushroom. Edible mushroom includes, button mushroom, oyster mushroom, king oyster mushroom, whereas reishi, lion's man, chaga, turkey's tail, cordyceps etc, are medicinal mushroom (Chang and Mshigeni, 2004). Some mushrooms are classified as poisonous like death cap, web cap, autumn skullcap, etc.

Fungi are well known for production of clinically important antibacterial and antifungal molecules like penicillin, griseofulvin, and cyclosporine. Among all the diverse fungi, mushroom which particularly belongs to Basidiomycetes are vast sources of bioactive molecules and other therapeutic uses. Till date almost 700 species of Basidiomycetes have been reported having some medicinal properties (Wasser, 2002). In recent few years, extensive research studies on pharmacological activities on medicinal mushrooms have been explored in some Asian countries. Majority mushroom bioactive molecules were identified and its immunomodulatory effect was found out (Zaidman et al., 2005). However, in India there is limited mushroom has explored for their medicinal properties (Ajith and Janardhanan, 2006). Some mushrooms used traditionally like genera, *Ganoderma, Grifola, Lentinus, Trametes (Coriolus) Auricularia, Flammulina,* and *Tremella* were reported to have significant immunomodulatory effects (Wasser, 2002).

Mushrooms are well explored for their bioactive molecules either exopolysaccharide or terpenoids. Mushrooms are the unlimited source of polysaccharides which possess anticancer, antiviral, antioxidant and immune stimulating properties. At present the whole world is suffering from COVID-19 pandemic which was started in Wuhan, China and later spread to the whole world. Initially in March, India has a lower number of cases but at present it reaches nearly 5 million (covid19india.org). Although extreme research is going on to find out medicine and vaccines for coronavirus yet the whole world is not successful for the same. However, there are several foods which can improve immunity of patients and increase recovery rates of patients. One such food is mushroom which possess enormous health benefits. Hence, present paper elaborates the mushroom exopolysaccharide structure and their antioxidant and antiviral activities.

Exopolysaccharides (EPS)

Mushrooms produce exopolysaccharides as part of its cell wall. The components are composed of two major types of polysaccharides: one is a rigid 20 fibrillar of chitin (or cellulose); the other one is a matrix-like β-glucan, α-glucan and glycoproteins (Zhang et al., 2007). The major polysaccharides isolated from mushrooms are glucans, linked with either β-(1-3) and/or β-(1-6) D-glucan. These glucans are either linear or in branched form and possess a backbone composed of α- or β-linked glucose units. Some of the glucan molecules possess side chains attached at diverse positions (Zhang et al., 2007; Yang and Zhang, 2009). The basic structure is β-(1-3) D-glucopyronan with 1 to 15 units of β-(1-6) monoglucosyl side chains (Mizuno et al., 1995). The structure of naturally occurring glycans is so diversified that it is difficult to define a universal protocol for their analysis (Zhang et al., 2007). Some of the different types of EPS produced by mushroom are listed in Table 1. In comparison with protein, EPS possess more biological information due to their structural diversity.

The monomer present in EPS structure are generally identified by either from whole EPS, partially hydrolyzed EPS or completer hydrolyzed EPS or its derivatization. Techniques used for these monomer identification are HPLC, paper chromatography, gas-liquid chromatography-mass spectrometry, gas-liquid chromatography or NMR spectroscopy. Composition of these EPS may vary from homopolymer to heteroppolymers and also comprised protein, sulfate, amine or phosphate group. Hexose and pentose sugars like glucose, galactose, xylose, mannose, fucose, and rhamnose are present in EPS structure. Though the monosaccharide composition is the same, different fungi synthesize polysaccharide that varies in molecular weight. The rationale behind variation in molecular weight is due to different monomer chain present or side chain patterns of polysaccharides (Mahapatra and Benerjee, 2013).

EPS was extracted from *Tremella fuciformis* and phenol sulfuric acid method was used to determined sugar content, whereas protein present in EPS was determined by Lowery's method (Cho et al., 2007). They have evaluated the effect of different cultivation methods, i.e., stirred-tank and airlift bioreactor on EPS composition. They have observed that proteoglycan consists of carbohydrates (89.12%, 86.48%) and proteins (10.88%, 13.52%), respectively. Monomer in carbohydrates was identified by gas chromatography. It contained mannose (56.10 ± 0.41%, 51.48 ± 0.10%), xylose (21.67 ± 0.06%, 22.58 ± 0.61%) and fucose (19.60 ± 0.22%, 21.81 ± 0.89%). Similarly, Lima and coworkers (2011), have extracted EPS from *Agaricus brasiliensis*. Mushroom EPS composed of 58.7% of mannose, 21.4 % of galactose, 13.1% of glucose, 2.8% xylose and 3.9% of rhamnose.

Table 1 : Chemical structure of mushroom EPS (Vadnerker, 2017)

Sr No	Mushroom	Polysaccharide Type
1.	*Armillariella tabescens*	α-(1→3)-glucan
2.	*Amanita muscaria*	Linear α-(1→3)-glucan
3.	*Agrocybe aegerita*	α-(1→4)-; β-(1→6)-glucan
4.	*Agaricus blazei, Grifola frondosa*	β-(1→6)-; β-(1→3)-glucan
5.	*Grifola frondosa, Polyporus confluens, Pleurotus pulmonarius*	Xyloglucan
6.	*Pleurotus pulmonarius, Pleurotus cornucopiae, Ganoderma lucidum, Agaricus blazei*	Mannogalactoglucan
7.	*Flammulina velutipes, Hohenbuehelia serotina, Leucopaxillus giganteus*	Galactomannoglucan
8.	*Ganoderma tsugae*	Arabinoglucan

Media composition and carbon source also affect the EPS composition. Chimilovski and coworker (2011) reported that when *Grifola frondosa* grown in submerged fermentation in the flask on soy and sugarcane molasses, it produces EPS with different carbohydrates and protein ratio. Higher EPS (5.14±0.26 g/l) was produced when sugarcane molasses were used as a carbon source. They have found that monomer present in EPS were glucose (12.76%), fucose (22.94%), xylose (13.98%), mannose (11.73%), galactose (2.86) and arabinose (36.03%).

Zhang *et al.* (2011) worked on chemical composition and antitumor activity of alkaline soluble polysaccharide derived from *Inonotus obliquus*. They have determined carbohydrate content of extracted polysaccharide by phenol sulfuric acid method and protein content by Lowry's method. EPS contained 92.6% sugar and 7.2% protein content. They analyzed monosaccharide by GC analysis and reported that EPS possessed L-rhamnose, D-xylose, D-mannose, D-galactose, D-glucose and D-galacturonic acid.

Medicinal mushroom *Ganoderma* also reported to have higher EPS production and EPS possess antioxidant and anticancer activity. Mainly, *Ganoderma* EPS contain glucose, galactose, manose, arabinose as their monomers (Fragaa *et al.*, 2014; Kheni and Vyas, 2017). Similarly EPS from *Pleurotus ostreatus* M2191 and *P. ostreatus* PBS281009 contains glucose, galactose, mannose, and arabinose as EPS monomer (Vamanu, 2012)

Sood *et al.* (2013) worked on extraction and characterization of polysaccharide from *Ganoderma lucidum*. Extracted EPS was characterized by FTIR. They have reported that peak at 3377.8 to 3396.5 cm^{-1} which was a strong absorption peak, a small acromion in 2924.2 to 2925.1 cm^{-1}, some peak in 1635.8 to 1650.3 and 1372.5 to 1375.2 cm^{-1}. They have also noted a strong absorption peak in 1074.8 to 1075.3 and 1043.2 to 1045.2 cm^{-1} and weak peak in regions 891.0 to 894.8 cm^{-1}. From all the major and minor peaks carbohydrate structure was confirmed.

Su *et al.* (2013) worked on EPS from *Morchella conica*. EPS was hydrolyzed with trifluoroacetic acid to find out its monomeric composition. Hydrolyzed EPS was analyzed by HPLC and they have reported only D-mannose as monomer. Osinska-Jaroszuk *et al.* (2014) determined total carbohydrate content of the exopolysaccharides using the phenol-sulfuric acid assay with D-glucose as a standard. They measured protein by Bradford protein assay. They have reported that it contained 303 ± 1.29 mg/g carbohydrate, 61.2 ± 1.2mg/g reducing sugar and 22.6 ±0.07 mg/g protein.

Thus, different mushrooms produce different types of polysaccharide and even composition varies from species to species in the same genera. Hence, they also play a role in diverse genetic information and their phenotypic trait. These polysaccharides possess some immunomodulatory effect. They have high antioxidant, anticancer and antiviral activities. Some antiviral activities and antioxidant activity reported are present here.

Antioxidant Activity

Mushroom EPS possesses antioxidant activity and hence studied widely for in vitro as well as in vivo activity (Lindequist *et al.*, 2005. Kozarski *et al.*, 2015). Their anti-oxidative activity in eukaryotic as well as in prokaryotic cells is due to their reduction property, the ability of scavenging reactive species, ability to chelate Fe^{2+} and the increase of some enzyme activities. It also takes part in antioxidative processes, such as catalase, Superoxide dismutase (SOD) and glutathione peroxidase (Guo *et al.*, 2007; Kozarski *et al.*, 2015). Presence of hydrogen in polysaccharide has the ability to scavenge free radical ions (Tsiapali *et al.*, 2001). Anomeric hydrogen of internal monosaccharide present in EPS renders higher antioxidant activity to EPS over its reducing end monomers (Tsiapali *et al.*, 2001).

Table 2: Antioxidant ability by various assay of mushroom exopolysaccharides **(Keles et al., 2011)**

Mushrooms	Dry matter %	FRAP µmol/g	DPPH 1%	EC 50mg/ml
Agaricus bisporus	94.55	12171.43	67.86	19.51
Chlororhyllum rhacodes	93.75	17885.71	80.64	11.18
Macrolepiota procera var. procera	93.26	7457.14	90.07	7.91
Amanita rubescens var. rubescens	94.05	31814.29	91.31	11.35
Pleurotous dryinus	92.68	11600.00	50.74	24.71
Pleurotous ostreatus	93.20	2385.71	86.35	11.07
Boletus edulis	93.53	52957.14	93.18	3.95
Boletus pseudosulphureus	95.17	47528.57	90.82	7.88
Leccinum scabrum	93.71	23814.29	74.19	18.74
Suillus luteus	93.85	58528.57	97.96	4.76
Lepista nuda	94.82	12171.43	85.61	16.2
Lepista personata	94.04	8314.29	89.33	16.91
Lactarius piperatus	92.13	3528.57	52.60	24.12
Lactarius volemus	92.77	3171.43	62.28	21.37
Russula nigricans	93.89	23600.00	78.16	19.40
Russula vinosa	91.25	1985.71	72.21	21.26
Boletus erythropus var. erythropus	93.59	62771.43	90.32	9.26

Vamanu (2012) measured the radical scavenging activity of EPS extracted from *Pleurotus ostreatus* using ABTS and DPPH methods. He observed that EPS of the two strains showed a higher DPPH scavenging activity than the samples from intracellular polysaccharide (IPS). Exopolysaccharide and intrapolysaccharide produced by both mushroom possessed a strong antioxidant power for the ABTS radicals. Liu *et al.* (2010) carried out the antioxidant activity of polysaccharide extracted from intracellular of different *Pleurotus* spp. by DPPH method. He observed that IPS from *Pleurotus corncopiae* showed the highest free radical scavenging activity that is 20.5±1.7%.

Osinska-Jaroszuk *et al.* (2014) estimated antioxidant activity of the crude exopolysaccharides of *Ganoderma applanatum* by the 1,1-diphenyl-2-picrylhydrazyl (DPPH) assay. They have found that tested EPS exhibited relatively weak antioxidant properties. In compare with control, tested sample showed 20 % higher antioxidant properties. Liu *et al.* (2013) determined radical scavenging activities of the different fractions of *Ramaria flava* using the DPPH assay. They have noted that water fraction showed the highest potent DPPH radical-scavenging activity, followed by ethyl acetate fraction, ethanol extract, petroleum ether and n-butanol fractions.

Keles *et al.* (2011) carried out antioxidant activity from methanol extract of 24 different wild mushrooms by FRAP assay and DPPH assay. Results of DPPH assay showed that the methanol extract of *Suillus luteus* and *Boletus edulis* showed the highest scavenging activity 97.96 and 93.18% respectively. Whereas, FRAP assay showed that extracts of *Boletus erythropus* var. erythropus possesses the highest activity compared to other extracts. Similarly methanolic extracts from highest reducing power 62771.43 and 58528.57ìmol/g from *Boletus erythropus var. erythropus* and *Suillus luteus* respectively compared to other wild mushroom.

El-Zaher *et al.* (2015) determined free radical-scavenging activities of three endo polysaccharides fraction (FI, FII and FIII) extracted from *P. ostreatus* fruiting bodies using different concentrations (5, 10, and 15 mg/ml) of exopolysaccharide by using DPPH assay. The result showed that DPPH radical scavenging ability of *P. ostreatus* endo polysaccharides increased gradually by increasing the fraction and concentration. The FIII endo polysaccharide at doses 5, 10, and 15 mg/ml showed the maximum scavenging activity 83.1, 85.1, and 87.2%, respectively compared to the scavenging effects of the control ascorbic acid at the same doses 95.03%, 96.5%, and 97.0%, respectively.

Antiviral Activity

There are several reports showing antiviral activity of polysaccharide extracted from diverse mushrooms belonging to ascomycota and basidiomycota. Some extracted polysaccharides were modified to increase activity against viruses. These diverse class of polysaccharide inhibit the growth of poliovirus, herpes virus, HIV, influenza etc., In some cases polysaccharide doesn't have direct inhibitory effect on virus but indirectly it boost immune system and thus affect as antiviral or decrease the chances of infection.

Aqueous ethanol extracts and polysaccharide of *Agaricus brasiliensis* was tested against Polio virus type 1 (PV1) (ATCC VR-58) using MTT cytotoxicity assay (Faccin *et al.*, 2007). HEp-2 cells (ATCC CCL-23 cell line) was tested and revealed that the CC50 for the aqueous extract was 5000 µg/ml, 2302 µg/ml for ethanolic extract and 969 µg/ml for polysaccharide. Its virucidal test showed that none of it was able to inhibit virus infectivity. However, it affects adsorption of viruses when added during the infection process. Aqueous extract from *Agaricus brasiliensis* has the ability to inhibit cytopathic effect of Western Equine Encephalomyelitis virus (Sorimachi *et al.*, 2001). Ethanolic extract from its fruiting body had the ability to inhibit cytopathic effect after adsorption of polio virus. *Lentinula edodes* commonly known as Shiitake produced a polysaccharide that exhibited antiviral activity (Rincão *et al.*, 2012). Polysaccharide was found to inhibit virus replication of bovine herpesvirus 1 and poliovirus 1.

Table 3 : Antiviral activity of mushroom exopolysaccharides

Mushroom	Antiviral Activity	References
Agaricus brasiliensis	Poliovirus type 1	Faccin *et al.*, 2007
Agaricus brasiliensis	Western Equine Encephalomyelitis virus	Sorimachi *et al.*, 2001
Lentinula edodes	Herpesvirus 1 and poliovirus 1	Rincão *et al.*, 2012
Agaricus brasiliensis	Herpes simplex virus	Minari, 2011; Cardozo *et al.*, 2014; Yamamoto *et al.*, 2013
Agaricus brasiliensis	Herpes simplex type-2 virus	Razumov *et al.*, 2013
Ganoderma lucidum	Herpes simplex virus type 1 and 2	Eo *et al.*, 2000
Pleurotus	Herpes simplex type 1 and 2	Zhang *et al.*, 2004
Pleurotus ostreatus	HIV	Wang and Ng, 2000
Fomes fomentarius	HIV	Seniuk *et al.*, 2011
Inonotus hispidus	Influenza A and B viruses	Awadh Ali *et al.*, 2003
G. lucidum	Virus replication	McClure *et al.*, 1992; Liu *et al.*, 2004
Grifola frondosa	Enterovirus 71	Zhao *et al.*, 2016
Lignosus rhinocerotis, Pleurotus giganteus, Hericium erinaceus, Schizophyllum commune and *Ganoderma lucidium*	Dengue virus serotype 2 (DENV-2)	Ellan *et al.*, 2019
Pezizales	HIV-1	Pérez *et al.*, 2014
Xylariales	H1N1	Hazuda *et al.*, 1999
Hymenochaetales	Influenza A and B4	Ichimura *et al.*, 1998

EPS extracted from *Agaricus brasiliensis* showed potential inhibition of herpes simplex virus (Minari, 2011). Similarly its sulfated derivative also possessed antivirus activity against herpes simplex virus (Cardozo *et al.*, 2014; Yamamoto *et al.*, 2013). Razumov and coworkers (2013) have tested aqueous extract from mushroom against Herpes simplex type-2 virus. They have noted that when aqueous extract is given to mice, it protects mice from Herpes virus.

EPS extracted from *Ganoderma lucidum* comprised phenolic molecule hispolon and it inhibited the growth of herpes simplex virus type 1 and 2 using Vero cells (Eo *et al.*, 2000). Various EPS fractions were obtained from B-glucan extracted from *Pleurotus* (Zhang *et al.*, 2004). These fractions were concomitantly added with virus showed effective in inhibition of herpes simplex type 1 and 2.

Similarly a glycoprotein of *Pleurotus ostreatus* fruiting body possessed antiviral activity against HIV (Wang and Ng, 2000). HIV virus was inhibited by EPS from *Fomes fomentarius* mushroom (Seniuk *et al.*, 2011). This mushroom produced a melanin-glucan complex which possessed higher antiviral activity in rats in comparison to drug zidovudine. This glucan also showed antimicrobial activity against *Helicobacter pylori*. Virus replication can be inhibited by mushroom EPS. Influenza A and B viruses replication was inhibited by EPS extracted using ethanol from *Inonotus hispidus* (Awadh Ali *et al.*, 2003).

Grifola frondosa produced a heteropolysaccharide having 40.5 kDa molecular weight and having a 1,6-β-D-glucan backbone (Zhao *et al.*, 2016). This polysaccharide was able to inhibit Enterovirus 71 (EV71), a causative agent of hand-foot-and mouth disease. Virus replication was blocked upon its application along with suppression of viral VP1 protein expression and 32 genomic RNA synthesis. Ellan and coworker (2019) has evaluated antiviral activity against dengue virus serotype 2 (DENV-2). For this antiviral activity, they have selected *Pleurotus giganteus, Ganoderma lucidum, Lignosus rhinocerotis, Hericium erinaceus* and *Schizophyllum commune*. They have reported that mushroom extract can be used as anti-dengue molecules with less toxic side effect.

Polysaccharide-protein complex of mushroom exert antiviral effect by inhibiting viral replication or by increasing immunostimulating activity (Lindequist *et al.*, 2005). *G. lucidum* produced a polysaccharide that possessed higher antiherpetic activity in cells which were pretreated or treated during the viral infection, rather than post infection treatment (Liu *et al.*, 2004). McClure *et al.* (1992) also reported that sulfated derivatized polysaccharide prevent early phase of the viral replication cycle.

Coronaviruses cause serious health threats to humans and other animals. Coronavirus is known to produce either Severe Acute Respiratory Syndrome Coronavirus (SARS-CoV) or Middle East Respiratory Syndrome Coronavirus (MERS-CoV). Novel coronavirus19 (COVID-19) has currently affected nearly 3 crore worldwide. There is no specific medicine yet discovered for it. However, patients are given vitamin C, Vitamin D, golden milk and healthy food to increase immunity. As mushroom EPS possesses antiviral activity it is beneficial to add it in a routine diet to build immunity and fight against coronavirus.

CONCLUSION

Mushrooms are very well known for their medicinal use since ancient times. It possesses antioxidant, antiviral, antimalarial and anticancer activity. It modulates the immune system and thus works as an immune booster. As discussed, many mushrooms possess good antioxidant activity and thus are able to scavenge reactive oxygen species and provide protection to cells.

REFERENCES

Ajith TA, Janardhanan KK (2006) Cytotoxic and antitumor activities of a polypore macro fungus, *Phellinus rimosus* (Berk) Pilat. *J Ethnopharmacol* **84** :157–162.

Awadh Ali NA, Mothana RAA, Lesnau A, Pilgrim H, Lindequist U (2003) Antiviral activity of *Inonotus hispidus*. *Fitoterapia* **74:** 483–485.

Cardozo FT, Camelini CM, Leal PC, Kratz JM, Nunes RJ, Mendonca MM, Simoes CM (2014) Antiherpetic mechanism of a sulfated derivative of *Agaricus brasiliensis* fruiting bodies polysaccharide. *Intervirology* **57:** 375–383.

Chang ST, Mshigeni KE (2004) Mushrooms and Human Health: Their growing significance as potent dietary supplements. The University of Namibia, Windhoek, Namibia.

Chimilovski J, Sascha H, Teixeira R, Thomaz-Soccol V, Noseda M, Medeiros A, Pandey A, Soccol C (2011) Antitumour activity of *Grifola frondosa* exopolysaccharides produced by submerged fermentation using sugar cane and soy molasses as carbon sources. *Food Technol Biotechnol* **49:** 359–363.

Cho E, Hwang J, Kim SW, Oh J, Yu B, Choi J, Song B, Won YJ (2007) Hypoglycemic effects of exopolysaccharides produced by mycelial cultures of two different mushrooms *Tremella fuciformis* and *Phellinus baumii* in ob/ob mice. *Appl Microbiol Biotechnol* **75(6):** 1257-1265.

Ellan K, Thayan R, Raman J, Hidari KIPJ, Ismail N, Sabaratnam V (2019) Antiviral activity of culinary and medicinal mushroom extracts against dengue virus serotype 2: an in-vitro study. *BMC Complement Alternative Med* **19:** 260.

El-Zaher EHFA, Hala AAM, Shalaby E, Attia WYF (2015) A comparative study on endopolysaccharides and exopolysaccharides production from some basidiomycetes with studying the antioxidant and antitumor effects of *Pleurotus ostreatus* mushroom. Egypt J Exp Biol (Zool) **11(1):** 1–14.

Eo SK, Kim YS, Lee CK, Han SS (2000) Possible mode of antiviral activity of acidic protein bound polysaccharide isolated from *Ganoderma lucidum* on herpes simplex viruses. *J Ethnopharmacol* **72:** 475–481.

Faccin LC, Benati F, Rincão VP, Mantovani MS, Soares SA, Gonzaga ML, Nozawa C, Carvalho Linhares RE (2007) Antiviral activity of aqueous and ethanol extracts and of an isolated polysaccharide from Agaricus brasiliensis against poliovirus type 1. *Lett Appl Microbiol* **45(1):** 24-28.

Fraga I, Coutinho J, Bezerra RM, Dias AA, Marques G, Nunes FM (2014) Influence of culture medium growth variables on Ganoderma lucidum exopolysaccharides structural features. *Carbohyd Pol* **111:** 936–946.

Guo XY, Wang J, Wang NL, Kitanaka S, Yao XS (2007)9, 10-Dihydrophenanthrene derivatives from *Pholidota yunnanensis* and scavenging activity on DPPH free radical *J Asian Nat Prod Res* **9:** 165-174.

Hazuda D, Blau CU, Felock P, Hastings J, Pramanik B, Wolfe A, Bushman F, Farnet C, Goetz M, Williams M, Silverman K, Lingham R, Singh S (1999). Isolation and characterization of novel human immunodeficiency virus integrase inhibitors from fungal metabolites. *Antivir Chem Chemother* **10:** 63–70.

Ichimura T, Watanabe O, Muruyama S (1998) Inhibition of HIV-1 protease by water-soluble lignin-like substance from an edible mushroom, *Fuscoporia oblique*. *Biosci Biotechnol Biochem* **62:** 575–577.

Keles A, Koca I, Gençcelep H (2011) Antioxidant properties of wild edible mushrooms. *J Food Process Technol* **2:** 130.

Kheni K, Vyas TK (2017) Characterization of exopolysaccharide produced by *Ganoderma* sp TV1 and its potential as antioxidant and anticancer agent. *J Biologically Active Prod Nature* **7:** 72-80.

Kozarski M, Klaus A, Jakovljevic D, Todorovic N, Vunduk J, Petroviæ P, Niksic M, Vrvic MM, Van Griensven L (2015) Antioxidants of edible mushrooms. *Molecules* **20(10):** 19489-19525.

Lima CUJO, Cordova COA, Nobrega OT, Funghetto SS, Karnikowski MGO (2011) Does the *Agaricus blazei* Murill mushroom have properties that affect the immune system? *An Integrative Rev J Med Food* **14(1–2):** 2–8.

Lindequist U, Niedermeyer T, Jülich W-D (2005) The pharmacological potential of mushrooms. Evidence-based complementary and alternative medicine: eCAM.2.285-99. 10.1093/ecam/neh107.

Liu J, Yang F, Ye LB, Yang XJ, Timani KA, Zheng Y, Wang YH (2004) Possible mode of action of antiherpetic activities of a proteoglycan isolated from the mycelia of *Ganoderma lucidum* in vitro. *J Ethnopharmacol* **95:** 265–272.

Liu K, Wang J, Zhao L, Wang Q (2013) Anticancer, antioxidant and antibiotic activities of mushroom *Ramaria flava*. *Food and Chemical Toxicology : an International Journal Published for the British Industrial Biological Research Association* **58:** 375-380.

Liu X, Zhou B, Lin R, Jia L, Deng P, Fan K, Guoyi W, Wang L, Zhang J (2010) Extraction and antioxidant activities of intracellular polysaccharide from *Pleurotus* sp mycelium. *Int Jo Biological Macromol* **47**: 116-9.

Mahapatra S, Banerjee D (2013) Fungal Exopolysaccharide: Production, Composition and Applications. *Microbiol Insights* **6**: 1–16.

McClure MO, Moore JP, Blanco DF, Scotting P, Cook GM, Keyner RJ, Weber JN, Davies D, Weiss R, (1992) Investigations into the mechanism by which sulfated polysaccharides inhibit HIV infection in vitro. *AIDS Res Hum Retroviruses* **8**: 19–26.

Minari MC, Rincão VP, Soares SA, Ricardo NM, Nozawa C, Linhares RE (2011) Antiviral properties of polysaccharides from *Agaricus brasiliensis* in the replication of bovine herpesvirus 1. *Acta Virol* **55(3)**: 255-259.

Mizuno T, Wang G, Zhang J, Kawagishi H, Nishitoba T, Li J (1995) Reishi, *Ganoderma lucidum* and *Ganoderma tsugae*: Bioactive substances and medicinal effects. *Food Reviews Int* **11(1)**: 151-166.

OsiNska-Jaroszuk M, Jaszek M, Mizerska-Dudka M, Blachowicz A, Rejczak T, Janusz G, Wydrych J, Polak J, Jarosz-Wilko³azka A, Kandefer-Szerszeñ M (2014) Exopolysaccharide from *Ganoderma applanatum* as a promising bioactive compound with cytostatic and antibacterial properties. *BioMed Res Int* Article ID 743812.

Pérez M, Soler-Torronteras R, Collado JA, Limones CG, Hellsten R, Johansson M, Sterner O, Bjartell A, Calzado M, Muñoz E (2014) The fungal metabolite galiellalactone interferes with the nuclear import of NF-kB and inhibits HIV-replication. *Chem Biol Interact* **214**: 69–75.

Razumov IA, Kazachinskaia EI, Puchkova LI, Kosogorova TA, Gorbunova IA, Loktev VB, Tepliakova TV (2013) Protective activity of aqueous extracts from higher mushrooms against Herpes simplex virus type-2 on albino mice model. *Antibiot Khimioter* **58**: 8–12.

Rincão VP, Yamamoto KA, Ricardo NMPS, Soares SA, Meirelles LDP, Nozawa C, Linhares RE (2012) Polysaccharide and extracts from *Lentinula edodes*: structural features and antiviral activity. *Virol J* **9**: 37–43.

Seniuk OF, Gorovoj LF, Beketova GV, Savichuk HO, Rytik PG, Kucherov II, Prilutskay AB, Prilutsky AI (2011) Anti-infective properties of the melanin-glucan complex obtained from medicinal tinder bracket mushroom, *Fomes fomentarius* (L.: Fr.) Fr. (Aphyllophoromycetideae). *Int J Med Mushrooms* **13**: 7–18

Sood G, Sharma S, Kapoor S, Khanna PK (2013) Optimization of extraction and characterization of polysaccharides from medicinal mushroom *Ganoderma lucidum* using response surface methodology. *J Med Plants Res* **7**: 2323–2329.

Sorimachi K, Ikehara Y, Maezato G, Okubo A, Yamazakki S, Akimoto K, Niwa A (2001) Inhibition by *Agaricus blazei* Murrill fractions of cytopathic effect induced by Western Equine Encephalitis (WEE) Virus on VERO Cells in vitro. *Biosci Biotechnol Biochem* **65**: 1645–1647.

Su CA, Xu XY, Liu DY, Wu M, Zeng FQ, Zeng MY, Wei W, Jiang N, Luo X (2013) Isolation and characterization of exopolysaccharide with immunomodulatory activity from fermentation broth of *Morchella conica*. *DARU Pharm Sci* **21**: 1.

Tsiapali E, Whaley S, Kalbfleisch J, Ensley HE, Browder IW, Williams DL (2001) Glucans exhibit weak antioxidant activity, but stimulate macrophage free radical activity. *Free Radic Biol Med* **30**: 393–402.

Vadnerker P (2017) Exploring exopolysaccharide from mushroom for their potential antioxidant and antitumor activity. Navsari Agricultural University, Navsari.

Vamanu E (2012) Biological activities of the polysaccharides produced in submerged culture of two edible *Pleurotus ostreatus* mushrooms. *BioMed Res Int* Article ID 565974

Wang HX, Ng TB (2000) Isolation of a novel ubiquitin-like protein from *Pleurotus ostreatus* mushroom with anti-human immunodeficiency virus, translation-inhibitory, and ribonuclease activities. *Biochem Biophys Res Commun* **276**: 587–593.

Wasser SP (2002) Medicinal mushrooms as a source of antitumor and immuno-modulating polysaccharides. *Appl Microbiol Biotechnol* **60**: 258–274.

Yamamoto KA, Galhardi LCF, Rincão VP, Soares SDA, Vieira TGP, Ricardo NMPS, Nozawa C, Linhares REC (2013) Antiherpetic activity of an *Agaricus brasiliensis* polysaccharide, its sulfated derivative and fractions. *Int J Biol Macromol* **52**: 9–13.

Yang L, Zhang L-M (2009) Chemical structural and chain conformational characterization of some bioactive polysaccharides isolated from natural sources. *Carbohyd Polym* **76(3)**: 349–361

Zaidman, Ben-Zion & Yassin, Maged & Mahajna, Jamal & Wasser, Solomon. (2005). Medicinal mushroom modulators of molecular targets as cancer therapeutics. *Appl Microbiol Biotechnol* **67**: 453-468.

Zhang L, Fan C, Liu S, Zang Z, Jiao L, Zhang L (2011) Chemical composition and antitumor activity of polysaccharide from *Inonotus obliquus*. *J Med Plants Res* **5**: 1251–1260.

Zhang M, Cheung PCK, Ooi VEC, Zhang L (2004) Evaluation of sulfated fungal b-glucans from the sclerotium of *Pleurotus* tuber-regium as a potential water-soluble anti-viral agent. *Carbohyd Res* **339**: 2297–2301.

Zhang M, Cui SW, Cheung PCK, Wang Q (2007) Antitumor polysaccharides from mushrooms: a review on their isolation process, structural characteristics and antitumor activity. *Trends Food Sci Technol* **18**: 4–19.

Zhao C, Gao L, Wang C, Liu B, Jin Y, Xing Z (2016) Structural characterization and antiviral activity of a novel heteropolysaccharide isolated from *Grifola frondosa* against enterovirus 71. *Carbohyd Pol 144:* 382-389.

Immunity Boosting Functional Foods to Combat COVID-19, Pages: 133–141
Edited by: Apurba Giri
Copyright © 2021, Narendra Publishing House, Delhi, India

CHAPTER - 11

BROCCOLI - AS IMMUNITY BOOSTER AGAINST COVID-19

Juthi Saha[1]*and Shruti Agrawal[2]

[1]State Aided College Teacher, Department of Food and Nutrition,
Prasanta Chandra Mahalanobis Mahavidyalaya,
111/3, B.T Road, Kolkata-700108, West Bengal, India
E-mail:sahajuthi@gmail.com
[2]Assistant Professor & Head, Dept of Food and Nutrition,
Budge Budge College, Budge Budge-700137, Kolkata, West Bengal, India
E-mail:shrutiagrawal74@yahoo.co.in
*Corresponding author

ABSTRACT

The World Health Organization (WHO) has declared the Corona virus (COVID-19) outbreak as a pandemic which has resulted in the greatest health challenge crisis and international communal health emergency in January, 2020. It is stressing everyone lives due to the potential to create detrimental overall effects and leaving deep and enduring scars. To fight this unprecedented situation, proper hygiene, sanitation, physical distancing, and food safety are at the priority list. COVID-19 spreads mainly directly or indirectly by droplets produced by coughing or sneezing of a COVID-19 infected person. So the time demands to boost our immunity using super foods, herbs, and supplements, etc. to fight against this deadly situation. Broccoli, a member of the cruciferous family, is a nutrient-packed powerhouse that can boost our immune system. It is a tremendous source of phytochemical including glucosinolates, sulforaphane, glucoraphanin, S-methyl cysteine sulfoxide, isothiocyanates etc. Moreover, it contains vitamin like C, E and K and minerals like iron, zinc and selenium. It confers desirable health benefits by providing antioxidants, regulating enzyme, apoptosis and cell cycle and reducing the risk of diseases including Type-2 diabetes. This paper aims to bring out the efficacy of these bioactive compounds present in this functional food so that common people can incorporate this in their diet to boost their immunity. Though any single food cannot claim to immune our system but its potentially high nutrients are silver lining against COVID-19 and it also paves the way for future research in this direction.

Keywords: Pandemic, Cruciferous family, Phytochemical, Immunity booster

INTRODUCTION

The Severe Acute Respiratory Syndrome Corona Virus-2(SARS-CoV-2) a novel fatal strain of Corona viruses has been declared as Public Health Emergency of International Concern (PHEIC) by the World Health Organization (WHO) on 11th March,2020 for creating havoc around the world (WHO,2020). This pandemic is the defining global health crisis of our time and the greatest challenge faced since World War II. It is stressing everyone lives due to the potential to create devastating all round effects that have obscured everyone's day-to-day dynamics.

COVID-19 is a multi-organ disease often associated with high morbidity. The symptoms of COVID-19 include coughing, sneezing, sore throat, fever, body and muscle ache (CDC,2020) and sometimes loss of smell and taste.COVID-19 spreads mainly directly or indirectly by droplets produced by coughing or sneezing of a COVID-19 infected person. Emerging data suggested that the peril for contracting corona virus infection is high under insufficient sleep, inadequate nutrition, physical or psychological stress, and other conditions that may adversely affect the body's immune system (Kalantar-Zahed, 2020). Corona virus mainly infects people with the low immune system as it becomes an open call for infections and other diseases like heart disease, cancer, diabetes and so on.

To fight this unprecedented situation, proper hygiene, sanitation, physical distancing and food safety are at the priority list. As till now, there are no preventive measures or vaccines developed to fight against COVID-19 but multiple pharmacological options are continuously being explored. So the time demands to boost our immunity using super foods, herbs and supplements etc. to fight against this deadly situation.

Plants are nature's gift to humankind. Plants are a promising source of nutrition as they not only provide micronutrients but also attribute bioactive compounds that help to boost the immune system (Mukherjee and Mishra, 2012). 80% of the population of developing countries depends on various plant extract for developing traditional herbal medicine for the treatment of chronic diseases (Owis, 2015) due to low economic condition. The list of plants having a possible role as neutraceutical is long but increasing demand has led to extensive pressure on the use of available resources.

American Cancer Society (1984) and National Research Council (1982) recommended incorporating various cruciferous vegetables, such as cabbage, broccoli, kohlrabi, cauliflower and Brussels sprouts in the diet due to its beneficial impact in the treatment of various diseases (Wolf *et al.,* 2015). Broccoli is a nutrient-packed powerhouse that can boost our immune system as it is a tremendous source of health-promoting substances like phytochemicals including glucosinolates, sulphoraphane, glucoraphanin, S-methyl cysteine sulfoxide, isothiocyanates etc. (Owis, 2015). Moreover, it contains vitamin C, E and K and minerals like iron, zinc and selenium. It confers desirable health benefits by providing antioxidant, regulating enzyme, apoptosis and cell cycle and reducing the risk of developing chronic diseases including Type-2 diabetes (Ma *et al.,* 2018).

This paper aims to bring out the efficacy of these bioactive compounds present in this functional food so that common people can incorporate this in their daily diet to boost their immunity. Though any single food cannot claim to immune our system but its potentially high nutrients is silver lining against COVID-19 and it also paves the way for future research in this direction.

Broccoli: the Green Beauty

Broccoli is scientifically known as *Brassica oleracea var Italica,* is a biennial vegetable of the cruciferous family (Jahan, 2010). It is originated from Italy but now it can be successfully grown in our country also. Broccoli is a cold-weather crop as it grows best when exposed to a temperature ranging to 18°C-23°C (Mukherjee and Mishra, 2012). Broccoli has dark green color flower heads and these flower heads are surrounded by leaves. These flowering head and small associated leaves can be eaten as vegetables.

Broccoli is exceptionally rich in phytochemical that possesses antimicrobial, antioxidant (Ravikumar, 2015) and anti-carcinogenic (Mukherjee and Mishra., 2012) properties. Broccoli is mainly composed of polyphenols, glucosinolates, isothiocyanate, sulforaphane and selenium (Samy and Gopalakrishnakone, 2010) and flavonoids, vitamins and minerals (Ravikumar, 2015). Broccoli is an exclusive source of glucosinolates and also a rich source of other health-promoting compounds including flavonoids, Sulphoraphane, isothiocyanates, hydroxycinnamic acids and other minor compounds (Owis, 2015). The presence of these substances in broccoli ensures great benefit to a human being by protecting against several forms of cancer and also shows pharmacological activities against various diseases. So, it can be regarded as Nutritional power house.

A balanced diet ensures a strong immune system that helps to withstand any assault against Severe Acute Respiratory Syndrome Corona Virus -2 through the expression of the gene, activation of cell and modification of signaling compound (Aman and Masood, 2020). The individual having a well-balanced diet appears to be safer with a better immunity system that lowers the risk of microbial infection and chronic diseases. A healthy diet is an utmost required to survive the current situation by strengthening the immune system. An adequate intake of iron, zinc, vitamin-A, vitamin-B6, vitamin-B_{12}, vitamin-C,vitamin-D is required to maintain a proper immune function (Yousafzai, 2013).

According to USDA (2014), broccoli is an abundant source of carbohydrate, potassium, Vitamin-K, Vitamin-C, Vitamin-A, Vitamin-E and folate and it is also a potential source of protein, dietary fibre, calcium, sodium, magnesium, zinc, iron and phosphorus.

Role of Bioactive Compounds Present in Broccoli

Bioactive compounds are extra nutritional substances that are present in small quantities in foods, mainly in vegetables and fruits and grains, which can modulate metabolic processes and provide health-promoting benefits (Santos *et al.*, 2019).

They are being extensively studied to evaluate the importance of human health. Broccoli is a predominant source of glucosinolates, sulforaphane and selenium and it also contains a negligible amount of indole glucosinolates (Mahn and Reyes, 2012). Broccoli sprouts are also rich in glucoraphanin (Vale *et al.*, 2015).

Glucosinolates, Glucophanin and Sulphoraphane

Glucosinolates (GLSs) are the nitrogen sulphur compound (β-D-thioglucoside-n-hydroxysulfates) which are predominantly found in broccoli (Ishida *et al.*, 2014). GLSs are not the functional bioactive compound of broccoli rather the hydrolysis product of GLSs by the enzyme myrosinase is the purported bioactive compound (Clarke *et al.*, 2011) which include isothiocyanates, thiocyanates, nitrites and oxazolidines. Among these, isothiocyanates have strong anti-carcinogenic activity (Guo *et al.*, 2014).

Glucoraphanin is an indirect antioxidant which makes broccoli a super food. It belongs to glucosinolates compound which are naturally present in cruciferous vegetables. These are converted into isothiocyanates by the enzyme called myrosinase which is also found naturally in cruciferous vegetables (Osman *et al.*, 2016). When raw broccoli is chewed, the glucoraphanin and myrosinase interact to create sulforaphane.

If glucoraphanin is consumed as glucoraphanin-fortified foods, beverages and supplements, a portion of it will get converted into sulforaphane by the human gut microflora. This is important because if broccoli is cooked for an extended period of time at high temperature, then the endogenous plant myrosinase enzyme get deactivated and thus the conversion become completely dependent on the gut microflora. This conversion rate varies from individual to individual as many type of metabolism is modulated by the microbiome.

Broccoli is also a potential source of sulphoraphane which induces Phase-I and Phase-II enzymes to detoxify cancer causing chemicals that help to prevent carcinogenesis and it also plays supplementary roles in preventing cancer by its anti-tumor action at the post-initiation phase (De Figueiredo *et al.*, 2015). In fact, sulforaphane has enduring antioxidant effects up to 72 hours compared to Vitamin C that only lasts up to three hours in the body. Sulforaphane is responsible for activating a rechargeable and sustainable antioxidant system in the body.

Role of Vitamin C

Since no pharmacological treatment against COVID-19 has come out till now, people are seeking ways to protect themselves. Vitamin C has a promising role in maintaining proper immune cell functioning. Consumption of Vitamin C less than or equal to 1gm/day reduces the mortality rate from common colds by 35% (Hemila, 2017). Broccoli is a rich source of Vitamin C and provides 89.2 mg of Vitamin C per 100gm (Mukherjee and Mishra, 2012).

Vitamin C has intense antioxidant properties that help in scavenging of oxidative substances that is why it is considered helpful in combating against SARS-COV-2 and other viral infection also. So, vitamin C need to be included in the treatment of COVID- 19. It also plays important role in the regeneration of Vitamin-E, normal neutrophils function, activation of pro-inflammatory transcription factor nuclear factor-kB, modulation of signaling pathways, regulation of inflammatory mediators, phagocytosis, gene regulation, signaling pathways in T-cells, increases neutrophil motility to reach the site of infection, activation of signaling cascade (Khan *et al.*, 2020).

Vitamin C should be included as a preventive therapy against SARS-COV-2 because studies showed that using early intravenous doses of vitamin C has a profound effect on the reduction of SARS-COV-2 infection. An oral dose of 6gm vitamin C plays a significant role in reducing the risk of viral infections (Kim, 2020) and also high intravenous doses of vitamin C is efficacious for the treatment of viral infections (Wang, 2020).

Role of Selenium

Selenium plays a vital role inimproving immune system especially by regulating oxidative stress processes (Rayman, 2012). It has been observed that low selenium status of the population is associated with susceptibility to COVID-19 and other RNA virus infections. The older population is more vulnerable to COVID-19 (Nikolich-Zugich, 2020) which is associated with serious clinical complications and mortality (Liu *et al.*, 2020).

Studies revealed that in the selenium-deficient environment, RNA virus becomes more virulent (Hiffler and Rakotoambinina, 2020). Evidence suggests that selenium aid in reducing oxidative stress by restoring selenoenzymes activities which include TrxR. The antioxidant effect of selenium helps to create a protective shield again the COVID-19.

Elderly people, especially with comorbidities are prone to selenium deficiency and oxidative stress have shown the worse outcome of COVID-19 (Cui, 2012). Selenium supplements help to significantly reduce viral infections. Sodium selenite (Na2SeO3) which is readily available and the addition of sodium selenium in the total parenteral nutrition solution help to increase TrxR activity (Broman, 2020).

The recommended daily allowance of selenium is 200 to 400 mg per day but approximately 600-1200 mg of sodium selenite for 2-3 weeks in hospital via parenteral nutrition solution is considered safe and effective against COVID-19 (Allingstrup,2015).

CONCLUSION

In the present scenario, the COVID-19 pandemic crisis has imposed a new set of challenges to maintain a healthy and productive life. The state of self-isolation, communal distancing and lockdown are significant measures to weaken the effect of the spread of the disease but these measures also harm an individual's life. People with low immunity are more vulnerable to COVID-19.

Consumption of a proper well-balanced diet can help to ensure an optimum immune function to battle the virus. This superfood is loaded with nutrients. So, it is sometimes also referred to as *"The Green Magic"*. Most of the people do not have the proper knowledge about the nutrient dense properties of Broccoli hence the intake is dismal in many parts of our country. This paper is an attempt towards creating awareness among the mass for better health and bright tomorrow.

REFERENCES

Allingstrup M, Afshari A (2015) Selenium supplementation for critically ill adults. Cochrane 566 Emergency and Critical Care Group *Cochrane Database Syst Rev*doi: 567 10.1002/14651858.CD003703.pub3

Aman F, Masood S(2020) How Nutrition can help to fight against COVID-19 Pandemic. *Pakistan J Med Sci* **36 (COVID19- S4):** COVID19-S121-S123.

Arshad MS, Khan U *et al.* (2020) Coronavirus disease (COVID 19) and immunity booster green foods: A mini review *Food Sci Nutr* **8(8):** 3971–3976

Broman LM, Bernardson A *et al.* (2020) Serum selenium in the critically ill: profile and supplementation in a depleted region. *Acta Anaesthesiol Scand* **64(6):** 803-809

Clarke JD,Hsu A, *etal*(2011) Bioavailability and inter-conversion of sulforaphane and erucin in human subjects consuming broccoli sprouts or broccoli supplement in a cross-over study design. *Pharmacol Res* **59(20):**10955-63

Coronavirus: Loss of Smell and Taste may Be Hidden Symptom of COVID-19— Business Insider. Available online: https://www.businessinsider.com/coronavirus-symptoms-loss-of-smell-taste-covid-19-anosmia-hyposmia-2020-3

Cui H, Kong Y, Zhang H (2012) Oxidative Stress, Mitochondrial Dysfunction, and Aging. J Signal Transductdoi: 10.1155/2012/646354

De Figueiredo SM, Binda NS, *et al.* (2015) The antioxidant properties of organosulfur compounds (Sulforaphane). *Recent Pat EndocrMetab Immune Drug Discov* **9(1):** 24-39.

Guo L,YangR,Guo Q, Gu Z (2014) Glucoraphanin, sulforaphane and myrosinase activity in germinating broccoli sprouts as affected by growth temperature and plant organs. *J Funct Foods* **9:** 70–77.

Hemila H (2017) Vitamin C and Infections. *Nutrients* **9(4):** 339.

Hiffler L, Rakotoambinina B (2020). Selenium and RNA virus interactions: Potential implications for SARS-CoV-2 infection (COVID-19). *Front Nutr* **7:**164

How Coronavirus Spreads, CDC (2020); (https://www.cdc.gov/coronavirus/2019-ncov/prevent-getting-sick/howcovidspreads.html?CDC_AA_refVal=https%3A%2F%2Fwww.cdc.gov%2Fcoronavirus%2F2019-ncov%2Fprepare%2Ftransmission.html.)

Ishida M, Hara M, *et al.* (2014) Glucosinolate metabolism, functionality and breeding for the improvement of Brassicaceae vegetables. *Breed Sci,* **64(1):** 48–59.

Jahan I, Mostafa M *et al*. (2010) Chemical and Antioxidant Properties of Broccoli Growing in Bangladesh. *Dhaka Univ J Pharm Sci* **9(1):** 31-37.

Kalantar-Zadeh K, Moore LW (2020) Impact of Nutrition and Diet on COVID-19 Infection and Implications for Kidney Health and Kidney Disease Management. *J Ren Nutr* **30(3):** 179–181.

Khan S, Faisal S *et al.* **(2020)** COVID-19: A Brief Overview on the Role of Vitamins Specifically Vitamin C as Im-mune Modulators and in Prevention and Treatment of SARS-Cov-2 Infections. *Bi-omed J Sci Tech Res* **28(3)**-2020.

Kim TK, Lim HR *et al*. (2020) Vitamin C supplementation reduces the odds of developing a common cold in Republic of Korea Army recruits: randomised controlled trial. *BMJ Mil Health,* doi:10.1136/bmjmilitary-2019-001384

Liu K, Chen Y *et.al* (2020) Clinical features of COVID-19 in elderly patients: A comparison with young and middle-aged patients. *J Infect* doi: 10.1016/ j.jinf.2020.03.005

Ma L, Liu G *et al*. (2018) Dietary glucosinolates and risk of type 2 diabetes in 3 prospective cohort studies. *Am J Clin Nutr* **107(4):** 617-625.

Mahn A, Reyes A (2012) An overview of health-promoting compounds of broccoli (Brassica oleracea var. italica) and the effect of processing. *Food Sci Technol Int* **18(6):** 503-514.

Miller S, Walker SW, et al.(2001) Selenite protects 465 human endothelial cells from oxidative damage and induces thioredoxin reductase. *Clin Sci Lond 466 Engl* **100(5):** 543 50.

Mukherjee V, Mishra PK (2012) Broccoli-an underexploited neutraceutical. *Sci Res Repot* **2(3):** 291-294.

Nikolich-Zugich J, Knox KS *et al*. (2020) SARS-CoV-2 and COVID-19 in older adults: what we may expect regarding pathogenesis, immune responses, and outcomes. *Gero Sci* **42(2):** 505 14.

Owis AI (2015) Broccoli; The Green Beauty: A Review. *J PharmSci Res* **7(9):** 696-703

Ravikumar C (2015) Therapeutic Potential of Brassica oleracea (Broccoli) - A Review. *Int J Drug Dev Res* **7(2):** 9-10.

Rayman MP (2012) Selenium and human health. *The Lancet,* **379(9822):**1256 68.

Samec D and Salopek-Sondi B (2019) Cruciferous (Brassicaceae) vegetables. In: Non-vitamin and Non-mineral Nutritional Supplements, NabaviSM(ed) and Silva AS(ed), Elsevier, in press, pp. *195-202*

Samy RP, Gopalakrishnakone P (2010) Therapeutic potential of plants as Anti-microbials for drug discovery. *Evid Based Complement Alternat Med* **7:** 283- 294.

Santos DI, Saraiva JMA, et.al (2019) Methods for determining bioavailability and bioaccessibility of bioactive compounds and nutrients. In Innovative Thermal and Non-Thermal Processing, Bioaccessibility and Bioavailability of Nutrients and Bioactive Compounds.Woodhead Publishing: Alpharetta, GA, USA, pp. 23–54

Shanghai Expert Panel, cited on Mar 23. http://mp.weixin. qq.com/s?__biz= MzA3Nzk5Mzc5MQ==&mid=2653620168&idx =1&sn=2352823b79a3cc42 e48229a0c38f65e0&chksm=84962598b 3e1ac8effb763e3ddb4858435dc 7aa947a8f41790e 8df2bca34c20e6f-fea64cd191#rd; 2020.

USDA(2013), Agricultural Research Service, *National Nutrient Database for Standard Reference Release 27.*

Vale AP, Santosa J, *et al.* (2015) Evaluating the impact of sprouting conditions on glucosinolates content of Brassica oleracea sprouts. *Phytochem,* **115:** 252–260.

Wang D, Hu B, et.al (2020) Clinical characteristics of 138 hospitalized patients with 2019 novel coronavirus-infected pneumonia in Wuhan, China. *JAMA* **323(11):** 1061-1069.

WHO Director-General's Opening Remarks at the Media Briefing on COVID-2020.(https://www.who.int/dg/speeches/detail/who-director-general-s-opening-remarks-at-the-media-briefing-on-covid-19—11-march-2020.)

Wolf S, Zikeli S, Fleck M *et al.* (2014) Building Organic Bridges **2:** 427-30

Yousafzai AK, Rasheed MA *et al.* (2013) Annual research review: improved nutrition–a pathway to resilience. *J Child Psychol Psychiatry* **54(4):** 367–377.

Osman AG, Chittiboyina AG *et al.* (2016)Chapter Three - Cytoprotective Role of Dietary Phytochemicals Against Cancer Development via Induction of Phase II and Antioxidant Enzymes. *Adv Mol Toxicol,* **10:** 99-137

Immunity Boosting Functional Foods to Combat COVID-19, Pages: 143–152
Edited by: Apurba Giri
Copyright © 2021, Narendra Publishing House, Delhi, India

CHAPTER - 12

PERSPECTIVE OF GREEN TEA: ITS IMMUNOMODULATORY ACTION AND HEALTH BENEFITS

Mansi Tiwari[1*] and Premila L. Bordoloi[2]

[1]Ph.D Scholar, E-mail: mansi4148@gmail.com
[2]Assistant Professor, E-mail: premilajmch13@gmail.com
Department of Food Science and Nutrition, College of Community Science,
Assam Agricultural University, Jorhat-785013, India
*Corresponding author

ABSTRACT

Tea, being the extensively consumed beverages around the world has numerous health benefits. It is consumed in varied forms namely black tea, green tea and oolong tea, determined by the post-harvest treatment and their chemical constituent. Owing to the fact that green tea is manufactured from unfermented tea leaves, they are a significant store house of a powerful anti-oxidant namely polyphenols and therefore are considered to be of comparative superior attributes. In general, green tea has been found to be of superior quality mainly owing to the fact that they are made from unfermented leaves and reportedly contains the high concentration of powerful anti-oxidant called polyphenols. Catechin derivatives are the most predominant constituents of green tea polyphenols which is responsible for the bioactive properties shown by green tea and are therefore have proved to be a potent contributor against various ailments including several types of cancer and numerous chronic diseases. The efficacy of green tea is spread to wide ranges including weight loss, hyperglycaemia, inflammatory bowel diseases, enhanced metabolism, skin disorders and hair losses. Recent studies have reported green tea components particularly epigallocatechingallate to have potential role in boosting immune functions. Clinical trials were performed to investigate the functionality of the extracts prepared from green tea in modulating immune responses by suppressing IgE production and induction of Tregs in experimental animals. With increasing interest in health and wellbeing there has been a significant rise in scientific investigations associated with health promoting action of green teaintake. Considering the above mentioned fact, the health benefits and immunomodulatory actions of green tea is reviewed in this section to have a clear understanding.

Keywords: Green tea, Immunity, Immunomodulation, Health benefits, Catechin, Flavonoids

INTRODUCTION

Tea, derived from plant *Camelia sinensis* is one of the most commonly taken beverages in the world. Based on the processing treatment involved, they are categorized into black tea, oolong tea and green tea. The preparation of green tea involves rapid steaming of freshly harvested leaves to inactivate the enzyme polyphenol oxidase and thereby preventing fermentation to get an unfermented dry and stable product. On the other hand preparation of black and oolong tea involves fermentation catalyzed by enzyme polyphenol. Oolongteaare produced by partial fermentation andblackteapreparation requires complete fermentation (Jigisha *et al.*, 2012; Gupta *et al.*, 2014; Botten *et al.*, 2015). The steaming operation performed during green tea processing allows enzyme destruction responsible for breakdown of color pigment thereby maintaining green leaf color during subsequent rolling and drying processes. In these processes the naturally intact polyphenols of green tea are preserved which contributes significantly in ameliorating human health (Cabrera *et al.*, 2006).

The health promoting potentialities of green tea is mainly attributed to its complex chemical constituents. Green tea comprises of polyphenols, alkaloids, caffeine, amino acids, carbohydrates, lipids, vitamins and other trace elements (Belitz and Grosh, 1997). Several Evidenceproves that green tea also consist of minerals such as Fe, Cu, Zn, Se, Na, Ca, Mg, Cr, Mn, P, Ni, K, F, Al etc. (Fernandez-caceres *et al.*, 2001; Corta *et al.*, 2002; Fung *et al.*, 2003 and Xu *et al.*, 2003). Among green tea constituents, polyphenols are the most pharmaceutically relevant compounds which plays a potent role in improvement of immune system functions along with the overall health and well being. Polyphenol concentration in dehydrated leaves is around 8–12 per cent (Min and Peigen, 1991; Graham, 1992; Katiyar and Elmets, 2001). Apart from polyphenols, gallic acid, kaempferol, myricetin, quercetin, caffeic acid and chlorogenic acid are also present in green tea (Graham, 1992).

The most pertinent polyphenol in green tea are flavnoids, of which catechin plays most promising role. Of the total water soluble constituents of green tea, catechin makes up around 30-40 per cent (Roowi *et al.*, 2010). Green tea comprises mainly of four main types of catechin which includes (-)-epicatechin (EC), (-)-epigallocatechin (EGC), (-)-epicatechin-3-gallate (ECG), and (-)-epigallocatechin-3-gallate (EGCG). Among these EGCG has been found in most abundance *i.e.* around 60 per cent while other catechin are less abundant in green tea. EGC makes up approximately 20 per cent of total catehin content in green tea followed by ECG with approximately 14 per cent and EC around 6 per cent. The catechin content of any particular green tea may also vary depending on certain factors (Ashihara *et al.*, 2010; Jigisha *et al*, 2012; Atomssa and Cholap, 2015). Apart from the type of tea several other factors such as portion of plant used, processing technique involved, geographical location, growing conditions, and tea preparation techniques influences the amount of catechins (Fernandez *et al.*, 2002; Lin *et al.*, 2003; Cabrera *et al.*, 2006). The chemical constituents of green tea marks several health benefits and possess anti-carcinogenic, anti-hypertensive, hypolipidemic, anti-inflammatory, anti-ageing and several immunomodulaory potentialities. Thus, in this chapter, an insight in different heath promoting efficacies of green tea is reviewed in details to have a better understanding.

Health Promoting Role of Green Tea

A linkage between green tea consumption and prevention of numerous health hazards has been evident since long. Several epidemiological evidences revealed green tea to be effective in lowering the risk of numerous chronic diseases (Zaveri, 2006). The efficacy of green tea lies in its catechin content more specifically EGCG which is a powerful anti-oxidant known for its role in controlling and preventing the growth of cancerous cells. It also performs hypo-cholesterolemic effect, inhibits abnormal blood clots formation, beneficial in cardiovascular disease (CVD), diabetes, obesity etc.

Anti-cancerous Role

Cancer involves uncontrolled cell division and tissue metastasis which are caused by a series of mutation. The anti-cancerous potentiality of green tea is depicted in many population based studies. This role is mediated mainly by EGCG. EGCG plays important role by inducing apoptosis and promoting cell growth arrest in cancerous cells. It modifies the signal transduction pathways that are majorly involved in proliferation, transformation, inflammation, apoptosis, and metastasis of cell (Khan *et al.* 2006; Na and Surh, 2006; Hu *et al.*, 2010). Green tea effectiveness is spread to prevention of skin cancer, hepatocarcinogenesis, lung cancer, multi-organ cancer etc. (Cao *et al.*, 1996; Katiyar *et al.*, 1997; Landau *et al.*, 1998; Umemura *et al.*, 2003).

Cardiovascular Disease Prevention

The beneficial role of catechin of green tea in preventing the risk of cardiovascular diseases has been proposed in varied studies. These beneficial roles are moderated by several mechanisms including anti-oxidant effects, endothelial function protection, lipid profile modification, anti-inflammatory and ant-proliferative effects. The anti-oxidative role of green tea is imparted by the ability of phenolic hydroxyl group to scavenge free radicals, thereby preventing oxidative modifications to LDL cholesterol. Green tea also proved to have a lipid lowering effect by reducing cholesterol absorption (Stangl *et al.*, 2006; Jochmann-Schiek *et al.*, 2008). In addition to this green tea also has vasculo-protective and anti-hypertensive effects which is mainly attributed to the activation of endothelial nitric oxide causing vasorelaxation and subsequently a decrease in blood pressure (Stangl *et al.*, 2006).

Anti-obesity

Green tea activity on obesity has received immense interest these days in the field of scientific investigations. Studies shows significant positive contribution of catechin present in green tea in influencing body weight and body composition (Kao *et al.*, 2006). The potential mechanism includes effects of catechin on thermogenesis and substrate oxidation, both of which are mediated by sympathetic nervous system activity. Apart from these several other mechanisms as modification in petite control, down regulation of enzyme involved in hepatic lipid metabolism and decreased nutrient absorption (Rains *et al.*, 2011).

In a randomized, double-blind, placebo-controlled, cross-over pilot study, 300 mg EGCG per day was given to six overweight men for two days. The investigation involved assessment of fasting and postprandial changes in energy expenditure and substrate oxidation. Results revealed no significant variations between EGCG and placebo treatments indicating, EGCG alone has the ability to ameliorate oxidation of fat in men and thus green tea being a rich source of EGCG can aid in anti-obesity effects (Boschmann and Thielecke, 2007). Other studies have also showed EGCG obtained from green tea to have anti-obesity effects. EGCG purified from green tea when fed to mice, resulted a decreased obesity in mice by modifying energy absorption and fat oxidation (Klaus *et al.*, 2005). Addtionally, caffeine and theanine were also effective in strengthening the effects of polyphenol on weight control of mice and its body fat accumulation (Zheng *et al.*, 2004).

Anti-diabetic

Green tea has shown its effectiveness in improving insulin sensitivity and reducing blood glucose levels. Green tea catechin have shown to inhibit carbohydrate digesting enzymes indicating decreased glucose production in gastrointestinal system thereby resulting reduction in glucose secretions. Several studies have also marked an association of green tea consumption to significant fall in plasma glucose and glycated haemoglobin levels (Rachel et al., 2009). From the study of Waltner-Law et al. (2002), it was evident that EGCG decreases glucose production of H4IIE rat hepatoma cells. In the study it was observed that EGCG mimics insulin, increases tyrosine phosphorylation of the insulin receptor and the insulin receptor substrate, and reduces gene expression of the gluconeogenic enzyme phosphoenolpyruvatecarboxykinase.

Immuno-modulatory Effect of Green Tea

The human immune system is complex and highly regulated internally. A healthy diet and lifestyle helps in normal functioning of the immune system, which may be altered by some diseases and medications. Bioactives present in tea, viz., Catechins, Theaflavins, Quercetin, Caffeine and Theanine can positively affect the immune system to bolster the body's natural response to infection. Green tea is known to play a vital role in modulating immune responses. Studies have shown that the role of green tea in immune-modulation is mediated both through innate and adaptive immune responses. The alkaloid caffeine of green tea has the ability to inhibit in vivo tumour growth by reducing tumour induced suppression of innate immune response (Mandal and Poddar, 2008). Green tea extract may also improve interferon secretions and phagocytic activity by boosting secretion of antibodies (Dona et al., 2003).

The potent component of green tea catechin plays vital role in presenting immono-modulatory responses. Prior studies conducted by Kim et al. (2006) on animal models showed EGCG to be beneficial in regulating inflammatory cell migration by suppressing MMP-9 production and by controlling free radical generation. Studies have also shown to modulate nitric oxide synthase activity in sensitized guinea pigs that counteract allergic asthma like reactions (Bani et al., 2006).

In a research investigation performed by Rahayu et al. (2018), green tea administration showed an improved immune response in rats infected by Candida albicans. In the study an immune-compromised condition was created in Wistar ratsby Dexamethasone 0.8 mg/kg and Tetracycline 12 mg/kg intraperitoneally for

7 days. A significant increase in the expression of IL-17A, IL-8, and HBD-2 in rats treated with green tea extracts showcasing its ability as immunomodulatory agent in an immunocompromised patient was seen in the study. The basic mechanism involved was that the IL-17A plays pivotal role in mobilization and activity of neutrophils which is an important component of innate immune system against infection. They are expressed by the activity of T helper cell 17 through RAR-related orphan receptor gamma t (RORãt) which results increase in neutrophils numbers resulting inhibition of oral candidiasis even in immunoompromised individuals (Etzioni, 2011; Dejima $et\ al.$, 2011). Green tea extracts also contain flavanoids that possessimmunomodulatory action, thereby enhancing the production of IL-2 which facilitates the proliferation and differentiation of T cellsto T helper cell 1 and 2. T helper cell 1 in turnsecretes various cytokines Interferon gamma (IFN-γ) to activate macrophages (Steinmann $et\ al.$, 2015). Flavonoid obtained from extracts of green tea also enhances proliferation of lymphocytes which could affect CD4+ cells to activate Th17 to produce IL-17A (Masatomo and Kazuko, 2014). This follows epithelial induction through IL-17R, to activate the synthesis of HBD-2, IL-8, and G-CSF. However in contrast deficiency of IL-17A leads to deficient neutrophil which enhances the risk of $C.\ albicans$ infection. Theepigallocatechin-3-gallate (EGCG) was found to prevent the TNF-α-induced cytotoxicity in ex vivo salivary gland cells (Hsu $et\ al.$, 2007). Saito $et\ al.$ (2015) in their study administered EGCG in Ten autoimmune sialadenitismodelofMRL-Fas-lprmice at an average dose of 592lg per day/mouse. The MRL-Faslpr mice treated with EGCG demonstrated an upregulated AQP5 expression on the APM of acinar cells through activation of PKA and inactivation of NF-kB, while IkB and HDAC1 played a pivotal role in the induction of AQP5 expression by PKA.

CONCLUSION

Green tea has been among the most widely consumed beverages in the world. Studies have also established green tea to possess numerous health benefits. It can serve as an important dietary components having potent therapeutic potential in the modification and control of various ailments such as cancer, CVD, diabetes, obesity and also possess immunomodulatory potentialities. Moreover, green tea can be easily affordable and can be served a multi-systemic strategy to improve health and well-being of individuals globally with relatively low hazardous adverse effects.

REFERENCES

Ashihara H, Deng WW, Mullen W, Crozier A (2010) Distribution and biosynthesis of flavan-3-ols in Camellia sinensis seedlings and expression of genes encoding biosynthetic enzymes. *Phytochem* **71(5-6):** 559–566.

Atomssa T,Cholap AV (2015) Characterization and determination of catechins in green tea leaves using UV-visible spectrometer. *J Eng Technol Res* **7(1):** 22–31.

Bani S, Gautam M, Ahmad SF, Khan B, Satti NK, Suri, KA, Qazi GN, Patwardhan, B (2006) Selective Th1 up-regulating activity of Withaniasomnifera aqueous extract in an experimental system using flow cytometry. *J Ethnopharmacol* **107(1):**107-115.

Belitz DH, Grosch W (1997) Chemistry of foods. Zaragoza: Acribia

Boschmann M, Thielecke F (2007) The effects of epigallocatechin-3-gallate on thermogenesis and fat oxidation in obese men: a pilot study. *J Am Coll Nutr* **26(4):** 389S-395S.

Botten D, Fugallo G, Fraternali F, Molteni C (2015) Structural Properties of Green Tea Catechins. *J Phys Chem* **119(40):** 12860–12867.

Cabrera C, Artacho R, Gimenez R(2006) Beneficial effects of green tea: a review. *J Am Coll Nutr* **25:** 79-99.

Cao J, Xu Y, Chen J, Klaunig JE (1996)Chemopreventive effects of green and black tea on pulmonary and hepatic carcinogenesis. *Fundam Appl Toxicol* **29:** 244-250.

Dejima T, Shibata K, Yamada H, Hara H, Iwakura Y, Naito S,Yoshikai Y (2011) Protective role of naturally occurring interleukin-17A-producing T cells in the lung at the early stage of systemic candidiasis in mice. *Infect Immun* **79(11):** 4503-4510.

Dona M, Dell Aica I, Calabrese F,Benelli R, Morini M, Albini A, Garbisa S (2003) Neutrophil restraint by green tea: inhibition of inflammation, associated angiogenesis, and pulmonary fibrosis. *J Immunol* **170(8):** 4335-4341.

Etzioni A (2011) Fungal infections: Blame the TH-17 cells. *Isr Med Assoc J* **13(9):** 561-563.

Fernandez PL, Pablos F, Martin MJ, Gonzalez AG (2002) Study of catechin and xanthine profiles as geographical tracers. *J Agric Food Chem* **50:**1833–1839.

Fung KF, Zhang ZQ, Wong JWC, Wong MH (2003) Aluminum andfluoride concentrations of the three tea varieties growing at Lantau Island, Hong Kong. *Environ Geochem Health* **25:** 219–232.

Graham HN (1992) Green tea composition, consumption, and polyphenol chemistry. *Prev Med* **21(3):** 334-350.

Gupta DA, Bhaskar DJ, Gupta RK (2014) Greentea:areview on its natural antioxidant therapy and cariostatic benefits. *Biol Sci Pharm Res* **2:** 8– 12.

Hsu SD, Dickinson DP, Qin H, Borke J, Ogbureke KUE, Winger JN, Camba AM, Bollag WB,Stöppler HJ, Sharawy MM, *et al.* (2007) Green tea polyphenols reduce autoimmune symptoms in a murine model for human Sjogren's syndrome and protect human salivary acinar cells from TNF-alpha-induced cytotoxicity. *Autoimmun* **40:**138–147.

Hu Y, Le Leu RK, Nyskohu, LS, Winter J, Young GP (2010) Combination of selenium and green tea improves the efficacy of chemoprevention of selenium and green tea alone in a rat colon cancer model. *J Gastroenterol Hepatol* **25:** 73-74.

Jigisha A, Nishant R, Navin K, Gautam P (2012) Greentea: a magical herb with miraculous outcomes. *Int Res J Pharm* **3(5):** 139–148.

Jochmann N, Baumann G, Stangl V (2008) Green tea and cardiovascular disease: from molecular targets towards human health. *Curr Opin Clin Nutr Metab Care* **11(6):** 758-765.

Kao YH, Chang HH, Lee MJ, Chen CL (2006) Tea, obesity, and diabetes. *Mol Nutr Food Res* **50(2):** 188-210.

Katiyar SK, Elmets CA (2001) Green tea polyphenolic antioxidants and skin photoprotection. *Int J Oncol* **18(6):** 1307-1313.

Khan N, Afaq F, Saleem M, Ahmad N, Mukhtar H (2006) Targeting Multiple Signalling Pathways by Green Tea Polyphenol-Epigallo-catechin-3-Gallate. *Cancer Res* **66:** 2500-2505.

Klaus S, Pultz S, Thone-Reineke C, Wolfram S (2005). Epigallocatechingallate attenuates diet-induced obesity in mice by decreasing energy absorption and increasing fat oxidation. *Int J Obes (Lond)* **29:** 615–623.

Landau JM, Wang ZY, Yang GY, Ding W, Yang CS 1998 Inhibition of spontaneous formation of lung tumors and rhabdomyosarcomas in A/J mice by black and green tea. Carcinog **19:** 501-507.

Lin YS, Tsai YJ, Tsay JS, Lin JK (2003) Factors affecting the levels of tea polyphenols and caffeine in tea leaves. *J Agric Food Chem* **51(7):** 1864-1873.

Mandal A, Poddar MK (2008) Long-term caffeine consumption reverses tumor-induced suppression of the innate immune response in adult mice. *Plantamedica* **74(15):** 1779-1784.

Masatomo H, Kazuko T (2014) Multiple effects of green tea catechin on the antifungal activity of antimycotics against Candida albicans. *J Antimicrob Chemother* **53:** 225-229.

Min Z, Peigen X (1991) Quantitative analysis of the active constituents in green tea. *Phytother Res* **5(5):** 239-240.

Na HK, Surh YJ (2006) Intracellular signaling network as a prime chemopreventive target of (–)-epigallocatechingallate. *Mol Nutr Food Res* **50(2):** 152-159.

Nursten HE (1997) The flavor of milk and milk products (I): Milk of different kinds, milk powder, butterand cream. *Int J Dairy Technol* **50(2):** 48–56.

Rahayu RP, Prasetyo RA, Purwanto DA, Kresnoadi U, Iskandar RP,Rubianto M (2018) The immunomodulatory effect of green tea (*Camellia sinensis*) leaves extract on immunocompromised Wistar rats infected by *Candida albicans*. *Vet World* **11(6):** 765.

Rains TM, Agarwal S, Maki KC (2011) Antiobesity effects of green tea catechins: a mechanistic review. *J Nutr Biochem* **22(1):** 1-7.

Roowi S, Stalmach A, Mullen W, Lean ME, Edwards CA, Crozier A (2010) Green tea flavan-3-ols: colonic degradation and urinary excretion of catabolites by humans. *J Agric Food Chem* **58(2):** 1296-1304.

Saito K, Mori S, Date F, Hong G (2015) Epigallocatechingallate stimulates the neuroreactive salivary secretomotor system in autoimmune sialadenitis of MRL-Fas(lpr) mice via activation of cAMP-dependent proteinkinase A and inactivation of nuclear factor κB. *Autoimmun* **48:** 379–388.

Stangl V, Lorenz M, Stangl K (2006) The role of tea and tea flavanoids in cardio-vascular health. *Mol Nutr Food Res* **50:** 218–228.

Steinmann J, Bauer J, Pietschmann T, Steinmann E (2013) Anti-infective properties of epigallocatechin-3-gallate (EGCG), a component of green tea. *Br. J. Pharmacol* **168:** 1059-1073.

Umemura T, Kai S, Hasegawa R, Kanki K, Kitamura Y, Nishikawa A, Hirose M (2003) Prevention of dual promoting effects of pentachlorophenol, an environmental pollutant, on diethyl-nitrosamine- induced hepato- and cholangiocarcinogenesis in mice by green tea infusion. *Carcinog* **24:**1105–1109.

Waltner-Law ME, Wang XL, Law BK, Hall RK, Nawano M, Granner DK (2002) Epigallocatecingallate, a constituent of green tea, represses hepatic glucose production. *J Biol Chem* **277:** 34933-34940.

Xu J, Zhu SG, Yang FM, Cheg LC, Hu Y, Pan GX, Hu QH (2003) The influence of selenium on the antioxidant activity of green tea. *J Sci Food Agric* **83:** 451–455.

Xu Y, Ho CT, Amin SG, Han C, Chung FL (1992) Inhibition of tobacco-specific nitrosamine-induced lung tumorigenesis in A/J mice by green tea and its major polyphenol as antioxidants. *Cancer Res.* **52**: 3875-3879.

Zaveri NT (2006) Green tea and its polyphenolic catechins: medicinal uses in cancer and noncancer applications. *Life Sci* **78(18)**: 2073-2080.

Zheng G, Sayama K, okubo T, Juneja LR, Oguni I(2004) Anti-obesity effects of three major components of green tea, catechins, caffeine and theanine, in mice. *In vivo* **18(1)**: 55-62.

Immunity Boosting Functional Foods to Combat COVID-19, Pages: 153–168
Edited by: Apurba Giri

CHAPTER - 13

APPLICATION OF PROBIOTICS AND FERMENTED FOODS IN IMMUNOSTABILIZATION

Subrota Hati[1*], Sujit Das[2], and Sandip Basu[3]

[1]Department of Dairy Microbiology, SMC College of Dairy Science,
Anand Agricultural University, Anand-388110, Gujarat, India
E-mail: subrota_dt@yahoo.com
[2]Department of Rural Development and Agricultural Production,
North-Eastern Hill University, Tura campus, Tura-794001, Meghalaya, India
E-mail: sujitdas557@gmail.com
[3]Department of Dairy and Food Technology,
Pydah College of Engineering, Kakinada-533461, Andhra Pradesh, India
E-mail: sansum_1974@yahoo.co.in
*Corresponding author

ABSTRACT

Probiotics are friendly bacteria and provide various health attributes to the human host. All the lactic acid bacteria and few yeasts are recognized as probiotic cultures after passing through probiotic tests *in vitro* and *in vivo*. Fermented milk prepared with dietary lactobacilli, preserves gastrointestinal micro-ecology and has therefore been used to treat a number of disorders in GI tract. Live and physiologically active lactobacilli have also been identified to have immunomodulatory implications. Specified lactobacilli species play an impactful positive role in host defence mechanisms, which may include regulation of invasive bacterial translocation and the production of specific and non-specific immune responses, or the production of short chain fatty acids, antimicrobial compounds. Colonization of the gut by lactobacilli has consistently been shown to stimulate the immune system and increase the host's resistance to infections. However, daily intake of probiotics in the form of tablets or through fermented foods may provide health benefits to the host by maintaing the native gut flora with good bacteria than bad bacteria and also provide the immunity to the human host.

Keywords: Probiotics, Fermented Foods, Immunostabilization, Lactic acid bacteria

INTRODUCTION

Probiotic Bacteria are "live microorganisms mainly Lactic Acid Bacteria having GRAS (Generally Recognized as Safe) status, that when ingested in our body in adequate amount (at least 10^7 cfu/ml or gm) can confer health benefiting effect to the consumer in the form of modulation of the inflammatory response, improving the nonspecific intestinal barrier, and reinforcing or modulating the mucosal and the systemic immune responses." Many types of lactic acid bacteria have long been recognised as therapeutic agents. Fermented milk intake, containing dietary lactobacilli, preserves gastrointestinal micro-ecology (eubiosis) and has therefore been used to treat a number of disorders of the GI tract. In several forms of host, dietary lactobacilli have also been identified to have immunomodulatory implications. Specified lactobacilli species play a positive role in host defence mechanisms, which may include regulation of invasive bacterial translocation and the production of specific and non-specific immune responses (Mrcp *et al.*, 2009).

Lactobacilli are gram-positive rods, usually non-motile, non-sporulating, micro-aerophilic, catalase-negative microbes, widely disseminated in nature and easily extracted from mammalian mucous surfaces, green plants, milk and fermented foods. In human system, lactobacilli are found in the mouth, lower intestine and vagina. Lactobacilli are also exploited for the manufacture of fermented milks like dahi, yoghurt, acidophilus milk, yakult, kumiss and bioghurt for human consumption. These products supply sufficient numbers of live dietary lactobacilli, which should be consumed live to achieve maximum therapeutic benefits. From this, concept of functional food has been evolved. Functional foods are those foods which give us health benefiting effects beyond basic nutrition. Probiotic fermented milk is considered as functional food and it has also the FOSHU (Food for Specified Health Use) status in Japan. Some Lactic Acid Bacteria (LAB) can also synthesize some essential vitamins like folate, Vitamin B12 etc. This is also considered as functional attributes of LAB.

Lactobacilli are known to produce several antimicrobial agents during milk fermentation, such as lactate, acetate, hydrogen peroxide and bacteriocins, that are potent against several intestinal pathogens, and hence the ingestion of these bacteria has been found to be helpful in controlling various intestinal disorders. They have also been found useful in recolonization of intestine after heavy antibiotic treatment and as a source of beta-galactosidase for lactose intolerants. Besides, they are effective in hypercholesterolemia, hepatic encephalopathy and tumorigenesis.

In addition to being an essential part of the gastrointestinal microecology of the host, lactobacilli also play a significant position in the immune protective system of the host by increasing specific and non-specific immune functions. Colonization of the gut by lactobacilli has consistently been shown to stimulate the immune system and increase the host's resistance to infections (Resta, 2009).

Health benefits by Probiotics include the following:

1. Improvement of the normal microflora
2. Prevention of infectious diseases and food allergies
3. Reduction of serum cholesterol
4. Anticarcinogenic activity
5. Stabilization of the gut mucosal barrier
6. Immune adjuvant properties
7. Alleviation of intestinal bowel disease symptoms
8. Improvement in the digestion of lactose in intolerant hosts

Desired Properties of Probiotic Strains

i) High cell viability, thus they must be resistant to low pH even 1.5 in stomach and bile acids up to 2%.

ii) Ability to persist in the intestine even if the probiotic strain cannot colonize the gut (continuous administration may be necessary)

iii) Adhesion to the gut epithelium (affinity towards hydrocarbon) to cancel the flushing effects of peristalsis.

iv) Also, they should be able to interact or to send signals to the immune cells associated with the gut.

Table 1: Different types of probiotics and their effects

Probiotics	Reported Actions
Lactobacillus acidophilus	1. Maintain balance of intestinal microflora
	2. Enhance immune response
	3. Act as adjuvant in H. pylori infection
Lactobacillus rhamnosus	1. Prevent antibiotic associated diarrhoea.
	2. Treatment of relapsing Clostridium difficile
	3. Anticarcinogenic action
Lactobacillus casei	1. Prevent intestinal disturbances
	2. Lower faecal enzyme activity
	3. Prevent superficial bladder cancer

[Table Contd.

Contd. Table]

Probiotics	Reported Actions
Lactobacillus acidophilus (NCFB 1748)	1. Lower faecal enzyme activity
	2. Reduce mutagenicity
	3. Prevent radiotherapy related diarrhoea
	4. Improve constipation
Bifidobacterium bifidum	1. Treatment of viral diarrhoea
	2. Maintain balance of intestinal microflora.
Lactobacillus reuteri	1. Colonization of intestinal tract
	2. Reduction of period of rota virus diarrhoea
Saccharomyces boulardi (yeast)	1. Prevention of antibiotic related diarrhoea
	2. Treatment of Clostridium difficile colitis

The Immune System

The mechanism by which the body recognizes accurately and specifically the foreign antigens and eliminates them is called immune system. It consists of number of organs and different types of cells. The organs of immune system comprise of bone marrow, thymus, spleen, peyer's patches and lymph nodes.

The immune system is commonly termed as an army and its various cells to soldiers. Their primary duty is to seek out and destroy or eliminate the invaders to protect our body. The function of immune system consists of two steps as follows: 1. recognition and 2. response. The immune system is able to differentiate between body's own cells and molecules from foreign molecules and cells.

All these cells develop from a kind of master cell, called hematopoietic (blood forming) stem cell and initially appear in the human embryo in the yolk sac. They, then, migrate to liver as the foetus develops. Blood cells are created in the liver of the foetus, but blood is normally produced solely in the bone marrow shortly after birth. These stem cells differentiate to form several types of blood cells, participating in immunity. These cells in general, are called leucocytes or white blood cells, which include granulocytes, monocytes, and lymphocytes. The granulocytes are subdivided into 3 groups called neutrophils, eosinophils and basophils. The neutrophils are essential in the host's defence against bacteria and some fungi, the eosinophils have a role in defending against parasites, such as worms and protozoans, while the function of basophil is less well understood. Monocytes (and related cells called macrophages) are crucial in the defence against intracellular parasites such as viruses and certain bacteria. Lymphocytes help in recognizing and destroying many types of pathogens. The T- lymphocytes give cell mediated immunity, while B- lymphocytes give humoral (antibody mediated) immunity (Erickson and Hubbard, 2007).

Several factors may decrease the immune function, including exposure to UV light, cigarette smoking, infection with viruses such as HIV and aging. Poor living conditions and malnutrition cause diminished resistance. Skin and mucous membranes in our body act in non- specific immunity by providing a physical barrier to invasion. Any damage to these barriers also decreases immunity. Microbial factors like the type and number of microflora on internal and external surfaces of body also affect the immune function significantly.

Host Immune Response

The mechanism of host's defence that keeps microbial parasites in check is called immune response. It is classified into two parts:

1. Innate (non-specific) immune response
2. Adaptive (specific) immune response

Innate Immune Response

This is first line of defence or immediate defence. Cell engulfs pathogen without caring what type of pathogen is and treats all pathogen equally. It consists of cells and proteins that are always present and ready to mobilize and fight microbes at the site of infection.

This is mediated by

i.   Phagocytic leukocytes
ii. Dendritic cells
iii. Specific type of lymphocytes called Natural killer cells
iv. Circulating plasma protein

Phagocytic Leukocytes

The body is protected against viruses and bacteria by these cells. Out of total leucocytes, 3 to 9% are phagocytes. These cells normally hunt foreign particles and then destroy them. Leucocytes that are phagocytic include Monocytes, Neutrophils, Eosinophils. Monocytes is type of WBC produced by bone marrow. They circulate in blood stream for about 1 to 3 days and then typically move into tissues throughout the body where it differentiates into macrophage and dendritic cells.

Macrophages or Dendritic Cells

Macrophages are protecting tissues from foreign substances. Phagocytosis is the process of uptake of microbes & particles followed by digestion and destruction of material. These are also capable of killing infected host cells using antibodies. Microbial fragments that remain after such digestion can serve as an antigen. This process is called antigen presentation and it leads to activation of T lymphocytes. These mount specific immune response against the antigen.

Neutrophils

Neutrophil granulocytes (often identified as neutrophils) are the most common type of white blood cells in mammals, accounting for 40% to 75% of total white blood cells. They are an essential part of the innate immune system. They're generated by stem cells in the bone marrow.

Neutrophils are phagocytes which are usually detected in the bloodstream. During the preliminary (acute) phase of inflammation, neutrophils are among the first inflammatory cells to travel towards the site of injury, particularly as a consequence of bacterial infection, environmental factors, and also some cancers. Chemotaxis is a process in which cells migrate from blood vessels to interstitial tissue in response to chemical signals like Interleukin-8 (IL-8), C5a, fMLP, and Leukotriene B4. They are the pus cells that predominate, accounting for their whitish/yellowish colour.

Neutrophils are activated within minutes of trauma to the injury site, and are the marker of acute inflammation.

Eosinophils

White blood cells and one of the immune system components responsible for battling multicellular parasites and some vertebrate infections are eosinophil granulocytes, generally referred to as eosinophils or eosinophils (or, less frequently, acidophils). They also regulate processes associated with allergies and asthma, along with mast cells. These are granulocytes that form in the bone marrow during haematopoiesis (the mechanism by which the body creates blood cells) before spreading into the blood (Kato *et al.*, 2005).

Functions of Eosinophils

- Activation of cationic granule proteins by degranulation.

- Reactive oxygen species (ROS) viz. hypobromite, superoxide, and peroxide (hypobromous acid, released by eosinophil peroxidase).
- Lipid mediators such as eicosanoids from the leukotriene (e.g., LTC_4, LTD_4, LTE_4) and prostaglandin (e.g., PGE_2) families.
- Enzymes, viz. elastase.
- Growth related factors viz. TGF beta, VEGF, and PDGF.
- Cytokines viz. IL-1, IL-2, IL-4, IL-5, IL-6, IL-8, IL-13, and TNF-α.

In particular, eosinophils also play a part in the combat against viral infections, which is noticeable in the accumulation of RNases in their granules and in the elimination of fibrin during inflammation. Eosinophils are key mediators of allergic responses and asthma pathogenesis, along with basophils and mast cells, and are correlated with the severity of the disease (Hogan et al., 2008).

Dendritic Cells

Dendritic cells (DCs) are antigen-presenting cells, (also known as *accessory cells*) of the mammalian immune system. Their main role is to process antigen content and introduce it to the immune system's T cells on the cell surface. They serve as messengers between the immune systems of the innate and the adaptive ones.

If activated, they move to the lymph nodes where, to initiate and form the adaptive immune response, they communicate with T cells and B cells. At certain development stages they grow branched projections, the *dendrites* that give the cell its name (dendron being Greek word for "tree"). While similar in appearance, these are distinct structures from the dendrites of neurons (Horiuchi and Weller 1997).

Natural Killer Cells

A type of cytotoxic lymphocyte that is essential for the innate immune system is Natural Killer Cells (or NK cells). In the vertebrate adaptive immune response, the function NK cells play is equivalent to that of cytotoxic T cells.

NK cells provide a quick response to virally infected cells and react to tumour formation, which occurs approximately three days after infection. Usually, MHC presented on infected cell surfaces is detected by immune cells, triggering cytokine release, initiating lysis or apoptosis.

However, NK cells are remarkable as, in the absence of antibodies and MHC, they have the capacity to identify stressed cells, accounting for a much quicker immune response.

Due to the obvious initial notion that they do not need activation in order to kill cells that are lacking "self" markers of class 1 belonging to the major histocompatibility complex, they were entitled "natural killers".

Primary and Secondary Immune Responses

Both humoral and cell-mediated responses are divided into two groups as follows: 1) primary and 2) secondary immune responses. Naive B and naive T cells are the B and T lymphocytes that have yet to recognize an antigen. When naive B cells come into contact with antigen, they multiply and split into two classes: the plasma cells secreting antibodies and the B cells of memory. The primary humoral response, which is the immune system's reaction to the antigen that the animal first encounters, is based on plasma cells. The primary response has a normal lag time where the naive B cells propagate and divide into plasma and memory cells.

Following that, serum antibody levels increase logarithmically, peaking around day 14, plateauing for a while, and then gradually declining as the plasma cells die. Memory cells are in the G0 stage and have a much longer lifetime than plasma cells; certain memory cells exist for the entire life of the organism. As a result, when the animal is exposed to the same antigen a second time, the memory cell population responds rapidly, triggering antibody secretion. The antibody levels peak in around seven days, and the antibody level is about 100 to 1000 times greater than the primary response.

A secondary immune response occurs when an animal's immune system responds to an antigen for the second time. Likewise, distinct mature T lymphocytes recognize an antigen-MHC complex, which causes them to proliferate and differentiate into TH cells, CTLs, and memory cells. The primary immune response is generated by effector cells, which is slower than the faster response given by memory T cells.

Lymphocytes

One of the groups of white blood cells that contain antigen-binding cell-surface receptors is lymphocytes. They, along with antigen presenting cells (APCs), are responsible of generation of an effective immune response. Lymphocytes give rise to the following immunologic attributes: 1) antigen specificity, 2) diversity, 3) immunologic memory and 4) self/nonself recognition. There are two key variations of lymphocytes viz. B lymphocytes (B cells) and lymphocytes (T cells). The B cells mature within bone marrow, express unique membrane-bound antibodies or surface immunoglobulins (sIgs) and ultimately produce antibodies, the effector molecules of the humoral branch of acquired immunity. T cells, on the other hand, grow in the thymus gland, release a specific antigen-binding receptor on their surface known as the T-cell receptor, and gradually become helper or cytotoxic T cells; the latter form the basis of the cell-mediated branch of acquired immunity.

B cells

B lymphocytes are a form of lymphocyte in the adaptive immune system's humoral immunity. B cells can be distinguished from other lymphocytes, such as T cells and natural killer cells, by the appearance of a protein called a B cell receptor on their outer surface. This specialised receptor protein makes it possible for a B cell to bind to a particular antigen.

The principal functions of B cells are to make antibodies against antigens, to perform the role of antigen-presenting cells (APCs), and to develop into memory B cells after activation by antigen interaction. They produce large amounts of antibodies in reaction to pathogens which then nullify foreign bodies such as bacteria and viruses.

T cells

T lymphocytes are a category of lymphocyte, a form of white blood cell that play an important role in cell-mediated immunity. They can be identified by the presence of a T-cell receptor (TCR) on the cell surface from other lymphocytes, such as B cells and natural killer cells (NK cells). They are named T cells since in the thymus, they evolve (although some mature in the tonsils). There are several subsets of T cells, each with a distinct function.

Two variations of T cells

1. **T helper cell:** Produce cytokines that direct the immune response.
2. **Cytotoxic T cells:** Produce toxic granules that contain powerful enzymes which induce the death of pathogen infected cells.

T cells and B cells are responsible for identifying specific "non-self" antigens during the antigen presentation process. When an invader has been detected, the cells produce complex responses designed to remove specific pathogens or pathogen-infected cells to the full degree. B cells respond to pathogens by producing large quantities of antibodies which then neutralize foreign objects like bacteria and viruses. In response to pathogens some T cells, called T helper cells, produce cytokines that direct the immune response, while other T cells, called cytotoxic T cells, produce toxic granules that contain powerful enzymes which induce the death of pathogen-infected cells.

B Cell Activation

It begins when antigen binds to cell-surface antibody molecules of a naive B cell. Some of the antigen molecules are internalized by the process of receptor-mediated endocytosis. These antigen molecules are combined with MHC class II molecules and processed and released on the layer of B cells. The antigen-MHC II complex is recognized by specific T_H cells, whose TCR binds to the antigen so presented. To proliferate and divide into memory B cells and plasma cells, the T_H cells activate the B cells. This activation is brought about by an interaction between CD40 of B cells with the CD40L of T_H cells. The T_H cells themselves are not activated since resting B cells lack B7 on their surface (B7 is present only on the surface of activated B cells). Most antigens activate B cells following this mode; these antigens are called thymus-dependent antigens and they generate immunologic memory.

There are two types (Type I and Type 2) of thymus-independent antigens that activate B cells without the help of T_H cells. Type 1 antigens activate a substantial proportion of B cell pool polyclonally when they are used at a high enough concentration. Such antigens bind to a B cell surface molecule that bypasses some of the early steps in specific B cell activation. An example of such an antigen are bacterial lipopolysaccharides. The Type 2 antigens are linear antigens that have appropriately spaced, highly repeating epitoe and are not readily degraded. Examples of such antigens are ficoll, D-amino acid polymers, Pneumococcus polysaccharide and polyvinyl pyrrolidone. Their repeating epitope cross-links sIg molecules in an antigen-specific manner, this cross-linking causes B cell activation.

Antibodies

Antibodies belong to a special category of proteins, called immunoglobulins (Igs) that is ordinarily glycosylated, is produced in animals in response to specific molecules, called antigens, and exhibits a highly specific antigen-antibody interaction. Each antibody specifically interacts with the antigen that had induced its production.

Antibody Structure

An antibody molecule comprises of two similar light chains (each chain containing 220 amino acids) and two similar heavy chains (each chain containing 440-450 amino acids), which are kept together through disulfide bridges; this constitutes the monomeric form of antibody. The variable region, designated as V_L and V_H respectively, is made up of about 100 amino acid long amino-terminal ends of both light and heavy chains. The amino acid sequence of this region differs among antibodies pertaining to particular antigens. The subsequent regions of the heavy and light chains are referred to as the constant region (classified as C_H and C_L, respectively) because the amino acid sequence of this region is nearly identical among antibodies of the same class. The variable region of each chain, in fact, contains 3 highly variable regions called hypervariable regions and denoted as CDR1, CDR2 and CDR3 (CDR= complementary determining region) separated by 4 invariant regions called framework regions (designated as FR1, FR2, FR3, FR4).

Probable Mechanisms for Host-probiotic Immunomodulation

➢ **Mechanisms of Action of Probiotics**
- Reduces luminal pH
- Releases antimicrobial peptides
- Prevention bacterial invasion
- Inhibiting bacterial attachment to epithelial cells

➢ **Enhancement of Barrier Function**
- Maximizes production of mucus
- Improves barrier integrity

➢ **Immunomodulation**
Enhances the function of:
- epithelial cells
- dendritic cells
- monocytes/macrophage
- lymphocytes viz. B lymphocytes, NK cells, T cells

Beneficial bacteria consumption strengthens intestinal mucous membrane immunity as well as overall body immunity by enhancing phagocytic activity and increasing antibody and lymphocyte development (Galdeano *et al.*, 2007).

The first line of defence against intruders is the healthy bacteria that make up the gut flora. They adhere to the intestinal wall and reinforce the physical barrier against pathogens. They compete with them for a spot to adhere on the intestinal wall and for the nutrients found there.

They also produce natural antimicrobial substances called bacteriocins. These two methods of defence discourage the implantation, growth, and survival of pathogens. The production of organic acids, hydrogen peroxide, and bacteriocins by lactic bacteria inhibits pathogenic activity. The organic acids produced by lactic bacteria regulate the intestinal pH to maintain it at a level that reduces the growth of infectious agents (Ruemmele et al., 2009; Kekkonen, 2008).

They can suppress pathogen adhesion by competitive exclusion, as demonstrated by Lactobacillus, Bifidobacterium, and Propionibacterium strains in in vitro models, and by triggering intestinal mucin formation, as demonstrated by Lactobacillus, Bifidobacterium, and Streptococcus strains in in vitro and small animal models. Antimicrobial agents such as organic acids, hydrogen peroxide, diacetyl, short chain fatty acids, and bacteriocins are also released by Lactobacilli and Bifidobacteria against pathogens. In mice and in vitro models, probiotics such as VSL#3 probiotic mixture, E. coli Nissle, and L. rhamnosus GG could improve the mucosal barrier system. Normalization of gut permeability, restoration of epithelial cells, and reinforcing of tight junctions may all contribute to improved mucosal barrier function, as seen in the rat model of L. rhamnosus GG and the in vitro model of E. coli Nissle.

Inflammatory mechanisms can also be influenced by probiotics viz., Lactobacillus and Bifidobacterium strains, through epithelial cells, and professional antigen-presenting cells, such as macrophages and dendritic cells, as reported in an in vitro model. In the Peyer patches of mice, macrophages have been shown to accumulate lactobacilli in a strain-dependent manner. Cytotoxic T cells and Th1 cells stimulate the cell-mediated immune response, which results in phagocytosis. In clinical trials with teenagers, Lactobacillus and Bifidobacterium strains increased phagocytosis and the number of cytotoxic T cells.

The activation of a Th1 immune response and low-grade inflammation in allergic children by L. rhamnosus GG has been suggested as a mode of action for preventing atopic diseases. The synthesis of IgA by mucosal lymphoid cells has been controlled by Bifidobacterium and Lactobacillus strains. In patients with Crohn's disease and infants, L. rhamnosus GG improved antibody-secreting cells, as well as faecal IgA in allergic children and Bifidobacterium in healthy children. Furthermore, in children, a composition of L. rhamnosus GG and B. animalis ssp. lactis Bb12 increased IgA-secreting cells. In a mouse model, L.

rhamnosus GG and *B. animalis* ssp. lactis Bb12 modulated the development of regulatory T cells, which regulate inflammatory and immune responses. Other than cytokines, probiotics can influence the development of inflammatory mediators. As shown in rat and in vitro models, initiation of low-level NO synthesis can be implicated in *Lactobacillus* strains' defensive behavior in the gastrointestinal tract.

Table 2: Effect of probiotic on innate immune system

Immune system effect	Organism
Improved phagocytosis capacity	*L. acidophilus (johnsonii) La1, L. casei, B. lactis Bb12, B. lactis HN019, L. rhamnosus GG, L. rhamnosus HN001*
Amplified NK cell activity	*L. rhamnosus HN001, B. lactis HN109 L. casei subsp. casei + dextran*
Triggered of IgA production	*B. bifidum L. acidophilus (johnsonii) La1, L. casei rhamnosus GG, B. lactis Bb12*
Lymphocyte proliferation inhibition and apoptosis promotion	*L. rhamnosus GG, L. casei GG B. lactis, L. acidophilus, L. delbrueckii subsp. Bulgaricus, S. thermophilus L. paracasei, E. coli Nissle 1917*
Raised cell- mediated immunity	*L. casei Shirota*

Table 3: Effect of Probiotic on adaptive immune system

Organism	Effect
L. rhamnosus	↓ Proliferation and activation of T cells
L. reuteri	↓ IL-12, IL-6, TNF-a, restricts the proliferation of B7.2, triggers regulatory T cell differentiation
L. casei subsp. alactus	↑ IL-12, IL-6, TNF-a
VSL #3	↓ DC maturation, "! lymphocyte proliferation, ↑ IL- 12, ↓ IL-10, ↑ Th1
B. longum	↓ IL-10, IL-12
L. casei	Induces regulatory T cell differentiation
L. gasseri, L. johnsonii and L. Reuteri	↓ IL-12 and IL-18, but not IL-10
L. casei	↓ IL-12 via macrophages stimulation

Table 4: Probiotic modulation of humoral immunity

Organism	Applied Species	Assessment Effect
Lactobacillus casei Shirota, oral (heat-killed)	Rodent	§ Systemic antibody reaction to ovalbumin. § Suppressed splenocyte immunoglobulin (Ig)E in vitro and serum IgE
L. casei, oral (live)	Rodent	§ Infection and antibody development in undernourished animals. § Improved sIgA and lowered enteric infection
L. acidophilus 1 Peptostreptococcus, oral (live)	Rodent	§ Translocation of *Escherichia coli* and serum total anti-*E. coli* IgG, IgE and IgM. § Reduced translocation and amplified anti-*E. coli* IgM and IgE
Bifidobacterium bifidus, oral (live)	Human	§ Total IgA and response to polio virus Increased sIgA

Table 5: Effect of probiotics on human disease

Disease	Probiotic	Assessment	Effect
Asthma	*Lactobacillus acidophilus*, oral (live)	Serum IgE and IL-4 Lymphocyte propagation	No variations
Rotavirus infection	*L. rhamnosus GG*, oral (live)	Diarrhea Serum total IgA and IgM and anti-rotavirus IgM and IgG	Period of diarrhea decreased; Improved anti-rotavirus IgA

Antitumor Properties of Fermented Milks

Cancer is the term associated with a variety of disorders that are characterized by the abnormal growth of cells. The lactobacilli may fight against cancer by either controlling the intestinal putrefaction or retarding the activity of enzymes that convert procarcinogens to carcinogens or by activating the immune system. The activity of faecal β-glucosidase, β-glucuronidase, nitroreductase and azoreductase, which are the enzymes that turn procarcinogens into carcinogens, was found to decrease in acidophilus milk. Bogdanov *et al.* (1975) isolated a glycopeptide fragment from the cell wall of *Lb. bulgaricus* and termed it as blastolysin. This compound exhibited antitumour activity against sarcoma -180 and Ehrlich ascites tumour. The cured animals retained permanent immunity to their respective tumours. Ayebo *et al.* (1981) also separated antitumour component of yoghurt by dialysis. Mice infected with Ehrlich tumour cells showed 33 % reduction in tumour growth, when treated with this yoghurt dialysate for 7 days.

Table 6: Anticarcinogenic properties of fermented milks containing dietary Lactobacilli

Experimental host	Agent	Effect
Mice induced with intestinal tumour by dimethyl hydrazine	Yoghurt	7-10 days feeding inhibited development of carcinoma
Human with colon cancer	Lb. acidophilus	8 of 14 patients showed mean decrease of 43 % in β-glucuronidase activities
Mice infected with sarcoma cells	Scandinavian ropy sour milk	50-75 % inhibition of sarcoma cells
Healthy adults	Lb. acidophilus	2-4 fold reduction in faecal β-glucurinidase, azoreductase, nitroreductase
Mice	Lb. bulgaricus Lb. casei	Improvised β-glucuronidase and β-glucosidase action
Mice infused with Ehrlich ascite tumour	Yoghurt dialysate	25-30% reduction in tumour growth, in contrast to control

CONCLUSION

WBCs (White Blood Cells) are responsible for both the innate and adaptive immune responses. Ingestion of probiotics and fermented food enhance function of these cells that indirectly improve immune system. Ingestion of fermented food activate immune system that provide antitumour effect. Probiotics can help maintain the intestinal microbial environment and the permeability barrier of the intestine and strengthen systemic and mucosal IgA responses, thus encouraging the ability to combat intestinal mucosal barrier infections. A healthy human microflora's therapeutic ingestion of beneficial microorganism cultures (i.e., probiotic approach) offers significant potential for the treatment and prevention of health manifestations correlated with compromised functions of the gut mucosal barrier and sustained inflammatory responses.

REFERENCES

Delcenserie V, Martel D, Lamoureux M, Amiot J, Boutin Y, Roy D, (2009) Immunomodulatory Effects of Probiotics in the Intestinal Tract. Curr Issues *Mol Biol* **10:** 37-54.

Erickson KL, Hubbard NE (2000) Probiotic Immunomodulation in Health and Disease. Symposium: Probiotic Bacteria: Implications for Human Health. *J Nutri* **130:** 403S–409S,

Galdeano M, De Moreno de LeBlanc M, Vinderola G, Bibas Bonet ME, Perdigo G, (2007) Minireview: Proposed model: Mechanisms of immunomodulation induced by probiotic bacteria. Clin Vaccine Immunol **14:** 485–492

Hogan S, Rosenberg H, Moqbel R, Phipps S, Foster PS, Lacy P, Kay AB, Rothenberg ME (2008). Eosinophils: Biological Properties and Role in Health and Disease. Clin Exp Allergy **38(5):** 709–50.

Horiuchi T, Weller P (1997). Expression of vascular endothelial growth factor by human eosinophils: upregulation by granulocyte macrophage colony-stimulating factor and interleukin-5. Am J Respir Cell Mol Biol **17(1):** 70–7.

http://en.wikipedia.org/wiki/Dendritic_cell

http://en.wikipedia.org/wiki/Eosinophil_granulocyte

http://en.wikipedia.org/wiki/Neutrophil_granulocyte

Isolauri E, Sütas Y, Kankaanpää P, Arvilommi H, Salminen S (2001) Probiotics: effects on immunity. *Am J Clin Nutr* **73(suppl):** 444S–50S.

Kato Y, Fujisawa T, Nishimori H, Katsumata H, Atsuta J, Iguchi K, Kamiya H (2005). Leukotriene D4 induces production of transforming growth factor-beta1 by eosinophils. *Int Arch Allergy Immunol* 137 **Suppl 1(1):** 17–20.

Kekkonen R (2008) Immunomodulatory Effects of Probiotic Bacteria in Healthy Adults. Research and Development Helsinki, Finland

Mrcp SC, Hart AL, Kamm MA, Stagg AJ, Knight SC (2009). Basic science review: Mechanisms of Action of Probiotics: Recent Advances. *Inflamm Bowel Dis* **15 (2):** 300-310

Resta SC (2009). Effects of probiotics and commensals on intestinal epithelial physiology: implications for nutrient handling. *J Physiol* **587:** 4169-4174.

Ruemmele FM, Bier E, Marteau P, Rechkemmer G, Walker WA, Goulet O (2009) Review on Clinical evidence For Immunomodulatory Effects of Probiotic Bacteria. *J Pediatr Gastroenterol Nutr* **48:** 126–141.

Immunity Boosting Functional Foods to Combat COVID-19, Pages: 169–176
Edited by: Apurba Giri
Copyright © 2021, Narendra Publishing House, Delhi, India

CHAPTER - 14

IMMUNE-BOOSTING AND NUTRACEUTICAL APPLICATIONS OF WHEY PROTEIN: CURRENT TRENDS AND FUTURE SCOPE

Tanmay Hazra[1]*, Rohit G. Sindhav[2], Mitul Bumbadiya[3] and D. C. Sen[4]

[1]*Assistant Professor, Department of Dairy Chemistry,
College of Dairy Science, Kamdhenu University, Gujarat-365601, India
E-mail: tanmayhazra08@gmail.com*
[2]*Assistant Professor, Department of Dairy Technology,
College of Dairy Science, Kamdhenu University, Gujarat-365601, India
E-mail: rohitsindhav7@gmail.com*
[3]*Assistant Professor, Department of Dairy Chemistry,
College of Dairy Science, Kamdhenu University, Gujarat-365601, India
E-mail: mitulbumbadiya@gmail.com*
[4]*Former Professor & Head, W. B. University of Animal and Fishery Sciences,
Mohanpur Campus, Nadia-741252, West Bengal, India
E-mail: drdcsen@rediffmail.com*
Corresponding author

ABSTRACT

The integral relationship between diet and health is well established now these days; therefore the proper utilization of nutrient-rich residues from food industries for designing the value added products, is the basic target for the modern food industry. Whey, is an important dairy industry waste and has been categorized to be admirable nourishment with an assortment of bioactive components. Whey protein comprises 20% of total milk protein provides a biological activity that surpasses the properties of superior quality amino acids. These proteins are one of the very few ingredients shown to modulate immune function in both *in-vitro* cell culture studies and *in-vivo* animal models. Whey proteins have proved beneficial against a wide spectrum of life threating diseases like cancer, diabetes, hypertension, obesity etc. This protein is also very useful for the recovery of exercise-injuries or skin diseases from radiations. Apart from health beneficial effects, it has several functional activities like fat replacer and emulsifier. This valuable protein is proving to be an immune-nutrient and its dietary interference to tackle life threating disease like cancer or viral diseases like COVID-19.

Keywords: Milk, Whey Protein, Immunity system, Immunomodulatory

INTRODUCTION

Food is the fuel of human life that not only provides us basic nutrition but more over it helps to provide immune boosting effects that helps to fight against many diseases also. Beyond nutritional aspect, Japan first time recognized the medicinal properties of food (Lopez-Varela *et al.*, 2002). After that, researchers all over the world tried to exploit the effect of different food ingredients or food components as whole, on several communicable as well as non-communicable diseases. Nutrient from food directly correlated to immune system of human body (Ibrahim and El-Sayed, 2016). Ibrahim *et al.* (2016) also reported that deficiency of several or specific nutrients from foods leads to weakened immune responses. In human beings, nutrient deficiencies impaired the immune response. Nutrition directly influence the immunoregulatory cells like T lymphocytes cells- extremely responsible for maintaining the immune function in body.

What is Immune System?

It is a defense system, mediated by complex network of organs cells and tissues, to protect the body from impairment. This complex system is generally recognized as immune system of body. Immunity system can be classified as below (Ibrahim and El-Sayed, 2016)

Innate (non-specific) – The specific immunity system that any individual can acquire with its birth.

Acquired (specific) - Highly specific than innate immunity and it supplements and augments the protection provided by innate immunity. B-cells as well as T lymphocytes cells able to regulate immunoglobulin (Ig); therefore those are highly responsible for this type of immunity system in body.

Milk as Unique Source of Immunomodulatory Ingredients

Milk is the white ambrosia for human society from prehistoric time. It not only contributes the basic nutrition, but also contributes to health beneficiary effect due to presence of highly bio-available bioactive components. Different bioactive components are directly influence the immune function (Li *et al.*, 2014) of human body. The majority of immunomodulatory activity of milk has been dominated by milk proteins (casein and whey) (Ibrahim and El-Sayed, 2016). Based on the solubility at pH 4.6 (20°C), milk protein can be separated in to two groups. Under these conditions, casein proteins are precipitated, while the proteins that remain soluble are known as serum proteins or whey proteins. These whey proteins actively act as immunomodulatory ingredients to human body (Middleton *et al.*, 2003).

Different Fractions of Whey Proteins

Table 1: Functions of different fractions of whey protein

1.	β-lactoglobulin	Principal whey protein, consisting of major essential amino acids.
2.	α-lactalbumin	It is the second most abundant whey protein. It has significant anti-proliferative effects as well as protective effects on gastric mucosa.
3.	Bovine serum albumin (BSA)	Carrier of fatty acids
4.	Lactoferrin (Lf)	It is an iron-binding glycoprotein generally present in milk and colostrum. It possess antimicrobial, antiviral, immuno-modulatory and antioxidant activities *in vitro* as well as *in vivo* system.
5.	Immunoglobulins (Ig)	Major immune protein
6.	Other minor fractions of whey proteins are Lysozyme, Glycomacropeptides, Lactoperoxidase (LPO) Enzymes etc.	

All these whey proteins directly or indirectly affects or contributes the immune system of human body.

Effect of Whey Protein on Immune Defense of Human Body

Single mechanism can't solely elaborate the immune defense of whey proteins (Sharma and Shah, 2010); therefore different mechanisms have been identified and given in below-

1. Glutathione (GSH) is an antioxidant molecule and whey protein is able to synthesize Glutathione (GSH) (Tseng *et al.*, 2006); therefore, it has been observed that the whey proteins able to increase the level of Glutathione (GSH) level in different tissues (Khan and Selamoglu, 2019). This is the primary mechanism by the whey protein for boosting the immune-system in

human health. Glutathione (GSH) prevents human tissue and cells specially brain cells against free radical or UV light exposure (Tseng *et al.*, 2006). However, the effect of whey protein against different diseases like arteriosclerosis or cataracts has been recognized by different scientific studies (Sharma and Shah, 2010).

2. Immunoglobulin combats against diseases by increasing the passive immunity to the children as well as adults by promoting the activity level of the immune system (Kadam *et al.*, 2018).

3. Transforming growth factors is a growth factors usually present in both milk and colostrum (1–2 mg/L) and (20–40 mg/L) respectively. These growth factors usually plays an important role for integration of gastrointestinal tracks for newborn animals. It directly inhibits the proliferation of neutrophils; therefore strength up host immunity (Gupta and Prakash, 2017).

4. Bovine lactoferrin able to stimulate immune systems by regulating inflammatory cytokines like stimulates proliferation of lymphocytes, TNF-α (Gahr *et al.*, 1991).

5. Whey proteins directly regulates and decreases the pro-inflammatory cytokines (IL-1 beta: 59% and IL-6: 29%) that directly affects or enhance the immune system of our body (Luhovyy *et al.*, 2007).

Others Health Benefits of Whey Proteins

Anticancer

Different medical research confirmed that the whey proteins were very effective for cancer patients (Patel, 2015). Whey protein is one of the major source of Gluthonine that helps to detoxify potential carcinogens as well as it stimulate immunity (Kadam *et al.*, 2018). Few researchers explained that the whey protein able to prevent the growth of different types of tumors (Patel, 2015).

Anti-Diabetes

Whey protein hydrolysate directly inhibit the alpha-glucosidase enzyme which helps to control diabetes. Some scientific researchers observed that the whey proteins helps to maintain the glycemic index in human (Kadam *et al.*, 2018).

Wound Healing

Whey protein is very rich source of bioactive amino acids; therefore whey protein products often suggested by physicians for the treatment of surgery or burn therapy (Kargi and Ozmihci, 2006). Lactoferrin has very significant effect against different viral diseases including skin diseases.

Improve Heart Health

Whey protein consumption reduces heart disease including stroke by increasing impaired brachial artery flow-mediated dilation by increasing plasma amino acids level (Patel, 2015). It is also observed that the consumption of whey protein increases the level of antioxidant and maintain low density lipoprotein level in body which indirectly improves heart health indeed. (Sheikholeslami and Ahmadi, 2012).

Anti-Ageing

Whey protein is a very rich source of numerous branched chain amino acids; these amino acids are extremely helpful for activities of muscle tissue. Therefore, whey proteins have been proved extremely fruitful against ageing related problems (Kadam *et al.,* 2018).

Studies proved that supplementation of whey protein isolates are extremely helpful for maintaining bone health. It is observed that the whey protein able to suppress the bone resorption and increases femoral bone strength (Kadam *et al.,* 2018; Kato *et al.,* 2000).

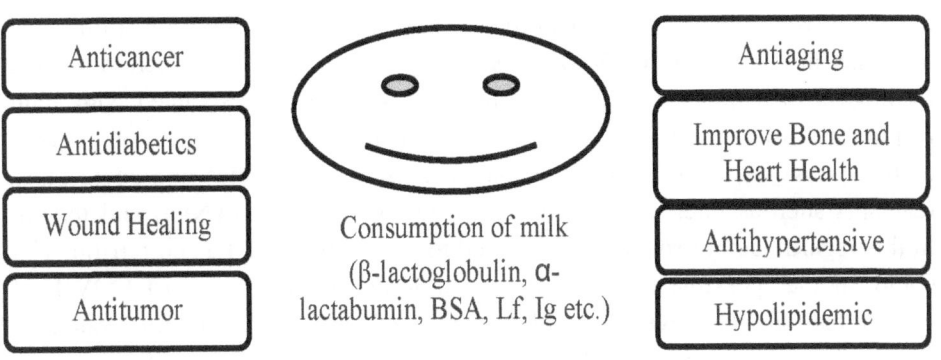

Fig. 1: Health effect of whey proteins

However, other health effects of whey protein including antihypertensive, antiviral, as well as antibacterial activities have been identified (Kadam *et al.,* 2018).

Applications of Whey Proteins in Food

Apart from health benefits, whey proteins used to play essential functions for modification the physic chemical as well as textural properties in different food systems, which is highlighted in below table (2).

Table 2: Typical function of whey protein in food system (Alfaifi and Stathopoulos, 2010)

S. No.	Functional Properties	Food System
1	Solubility	Beverages
2	Water absorption	Meat/Bakery
3	Viscosity	Soups/gravy
4	Gelation	Meat/fish
5	Emulsion properties	Infant formula
6	Fat absorption	Sausages
7	Foaming properties	Whipped topping
8	Flavour binding	Formulated foods
9	Mineral binding	Nutritional foods

Lactoferrin(Lf) a Potent Whey Protein Against COVID-19 Virus

Lf has been found to inhibit viral entry via binding to host cell surface of human corona virus. However, Nobel COVID-19 virus infections pathway is very similar to other coronavirus, so lactoferrin treatment could be potential against this virus too. The mortality from COVID-19 is not simply due to viral infection but is a result of a *cytokine storm syndrome* in selected patients- associated with acute respiratory distress and subsequent mortality. Due to this virus infection majority of the cases, has been recognized that increases in cytokines and acute phase reactants such as interleukin IL-6, tumor necrosis factor-a (TNFa) and ferritin. In this regard, lactoferrin has been proved to reduce IL-6, TNFa and ferritin. That could another possible mechanism of lactoferrin treatment against COVID-19 virus infections. However no published research has directly demonstrated the effect of lactoferrin on covid 19 disease but antiviral drugs along with lactoferrin supplement could be an alternative treatment against this pandemic.

CONCLUSION

Immune system is a complex bio-function of body, mediated by different tissue, cells or organs. More over this complex system is mediated by bio-chemical pathways mediated by numerous macro and micro biomolecules in body. However these extremely important bio-molecules are synthesis in body itself or those use to enter in body system through foods. So foods as whole or modified use to play an important role to maintain the integrity of immune mechanisms of body as such. Whey protein comprise almost 20% of whole milk proteins and comprises of different fractions such as all β-lactoglobulin, α-lactalbumin, immunoglobulin etc. All these sub-fractions use to play very effective role to immune modulating effects for human body with different mechanisms. Moreover, clinical studies proved the efficacy of these proteins against a wide ranges of diseases including cancer or deadly viral mediated diseases. Apart from health benefits whey proteins use to play a very important function for modification of different physic-chemical properties of different foods and beverages. However, bioavaibility of these proteins during processing is the main challenge facing by food researchers.

REFERENCES

Alfaifi MS, Stathopoulos CE (2010) Effect of egg yolk substitution by sweet whey protein isolate on texture, stability and colour of Gelato style vanilla ice cream. *Inter J Dairy Technol* **63(4):** 593-598.

Gahr M, Speer CP, Damerau B, Sawatzki G (1991) Influence of lactoferrin on the function of human polymorphonuclear leukocytes and monocytes. *J Leukoc Biol* **49(5):** 427-433.

Gupta C, Prakash D (2017) Therapeutic potential of milk whey. *Beverages* **3(3):** 31.

Ibrahim KS, El-Sayed EM (2016) Potential role of nutrients on immunity. *Inter Food Res J* **23(2):** 464-474.

Kadam B, Ambadkar R, Rathod K, Landge S (2018) Health benefits of whey— a brief review. *Int J Livestock Res* **8(5):** 31-49.

Kargi F, Ozmihci S (2006) Utilization of cheese whey powder (CWP) for ethanol fermentation: effect of operating parameters. *Enzyme Micro Technol* **38(3):** 711-718.

Kato K, Toba Y, Matsuyama H, Yamamura JI, Matsuoka Y, Kawakami H, Itanashi A, Kumegawa M, Aoe S, Takada, Y (2000) Milk basic protein enhances the bone strength in ovariectomized rats. *J Food Biochem* **24(6):** 467-476.

Khan UM, Selamoglu Z (2019) Nutritional and medical perspectives of whey protein: A historical overview. *J Pharm Care* **7(4):** 112-117.

Li M, Monaco MH, Wang M, Comstock SS, Kuhlenschmidt TB, Fahey JrGC, Miller MJ, Kuhlenschmidt MS, Donovan SM (2014) Human milk oligosaccharides shorten rotavirus-induced diarrhea and modulate piglet mucosal immunity and colonic microbiota. *ISME J* **8(8):** 1609-1620.

Lopez-Varela S, Gonzalez-Gross M, Marcos A (2002) Functional foods and the immune system: a review. *Eur J Clin Nutr* **56(3):** S29-S33.

Luhovyy BL, Akhavan T, Anderson GH (2007) Whey proteins in the regulation of food intake and satiety. *J Am Coll Nutr* **26(6):** 704S-712S.

Middleton N, Reid JR, Coolbear T, Jelen P (2003) Proliferation and intracellular glutathione in Jurkat T cells with concentrated whey protein products. *Int Dairy J* **13(7):** 565-573.

Patel S (2015) Emerging trends in nutraceutical applications of whey protein and its derivatives. *J Food Sci Technol* **52(11):** 6847-6858.

Sharma R, Shah N (2010) Health benefits of whey proteins. *Nutr Foods* **9(4):** 39-45.

Sheikholeslami VD, Ahmadi KGF (2012) Changes in antioxidant status and cardiovascular risk factors of overweight young men after six weeks supplementation of whey protein isolate and resistance training. *Appetite* **59(3):** 673-678.

Tseng YM, Lin SK, Hsiao JK, Chen J, Lee JH, Wu SH, Tsai LY (2006) Whey protein concentrate promotes the production of glutathione (GSH) by GSH reductase in the PC12 cell line after acute ethanol exposure. *Food Chem Toxicol* **44(4):** 574-578.

Immunity Boosting Functional Foods to Combat COVID-19, Pages: 177–188
Edited by: Apurba Giri
Copyright © 2021, Narendra Publishing House, Delhi, India

C H A P T E R - 15

BIOFUNCTIONAL PROPERTIES OF TRADITIONAL INDIAN FERMENTED MILK FOODS FOR IMMUNITY BOOSTING

Mahasweta Bhattacharyya[1], Chandrakanta Sen[2]*
and Pinaki Ranjan Ray[3]

[1]*M.Tech Scholar, Dept. of Dairy Chemistry,*
E-mail: mahaswetabhattacharyyadt1418@gmail.com
[2]*M.Tech Scholar, Dept. of Dairy Chemistry,*
E-mail: sen.chandrakanta10@gmail.com
[3]*Professor, Dept. of Dairy Chemistry,*
E-mail: pinakirray@gmail.com
West Bengal University of Animal and Fishery Sciences
Mohanpur Campus, Nadia-741252, West Bengal, India
*Corresponding author

ABSTRACT

Boosting immunity is the most important preventive measure to fight against different externally acquired infection like SARS- COV2 outbreak presently prevailing all over the world. Food plays a major role in enhancing immunity of the body. Fermented foods especially fermented milk foods are a great source of bioactive peptides that help in boosting immunity. India has a plethora of traditional fermented milk foods such as dahi, lassi, srhikhand, chhurpi etc. in its kitty which are having abundant biofunctional activities. They exhibit various health benefits especially immunomodulation, antimicrobial, antithrombotic and antioxidative properties which are mostly required to combat the detrimental effects of the pathogens. They are also a rich source of several vitamins and micronutrients required for boosting immunity. The present article focuses on the biofunctional properties of traditional Indian fermented milk foods which have the capability of enhancing immunity of the body. It also explores the way to fight against the SARS-COV2 virus by marinating proper immunity with simple available resources found in traditional Indian fermented milk foods.

Keywords: Bio-functional, Immunity, Fermented milk, SARS-CoV 2, Traditional, Bioactive peptides.

INTRODUCTION

Nowadays people are more cautious to their health. They prefer health beneficial natural products. For this consequence global demand for health-promoting foods are gradually increasing. Consumers are showing intereston bioactive compounds enriched foods like fermented foods, nutraceuticals, therapeutic foods, super-foods, functional dairy products, designer foods and probiotics etc. Presently foods do not recede only hunger but also boost up energy and develop health conditions (Gortzi *et al.*, 2015). Bio-functional foods exhibit physiological benefits, biological effects apart from nutritional quality (Mohanti *et al.*, 2017). Fermented milks are rich source of bioactive peptides which manifest bio-functional properties (Tamang, 2020). Bioactive peptides are mostly formed through enzymatic hydrolysis process or by fermentation with suitable microorganisms (Chakrabarti *et al.*, 2018; Hati *et al.*, 2015) and exhibit several physiological and biochemical activities like antidiabetic, immunomodulatory, antihypertensive, antimicrobial, opioid, cytomodulatory, antioxidative and antithrombotic (Mohanty *et al.*, 2016). Bioactive peptides alsohelp to cure diarrhoea, thrombosis, mineral malabsorption, dental carries (Pophaly *et al.*, 2018). Different traditional fermented milk products like dahi, shrikhand, lassi etc. exhibit biofuntional properties because of their bioactive peptide content (Haque *et al.*, 2008). Since ancient time, consumption of these fermented milk foods have been held responsible for probiotic activities (Tamang, 2020). Indian traditional fermented milk foods have attracted attention in the recent Covid-19 pandemic situation in view of its capability of boosting up immune system. Present article is focused on introducingtraditional fermentedmilk foods available in different states of India which are capable of enhancing our immunity with their potential bio-functional properties.

Indian Traditional Fermented Dairy Products

India is a tropical country with an average temperatureof 25-31°C. The ancient people of India started to preserve the food at this high temperature with the help of the fermentation process. This preservation technique resulted to produce new nutritious foods which were reported to be healthy. Dahi is one of the earliest fermented dairy products of the Hindus mentioned in Upanishad and Veda. Buttermilk, dahi, ghee (from fermented butter) were consumed extensively during 3000 BC. The by-products of butter are buttermilk, mostly consumed as a non-alcoholic beverage. Misti dahi is very famous among Bengalis as a sweetened fermented dairy product. Shrikhand is a fermented sweet viscous dessert popular in Gujarat, Rajasthan, and Haryana. Chhurpi is a yak milk cheese variety famous in Arunachal Pradesh. Fermented milk foods such as Somar, Phuh or Azaco cheese, Bandel cheese, Mohi, Gheu, Mattha, Rabadi, Chilika etc. are available in different states of India but not so much familiar to us. These lesser known products also exhibit health benefits as they contain similar types of cultures used in popular fermented milk products. Different types of traditional fermented milk products foundacross the states of India are presented in **Fig.1.**

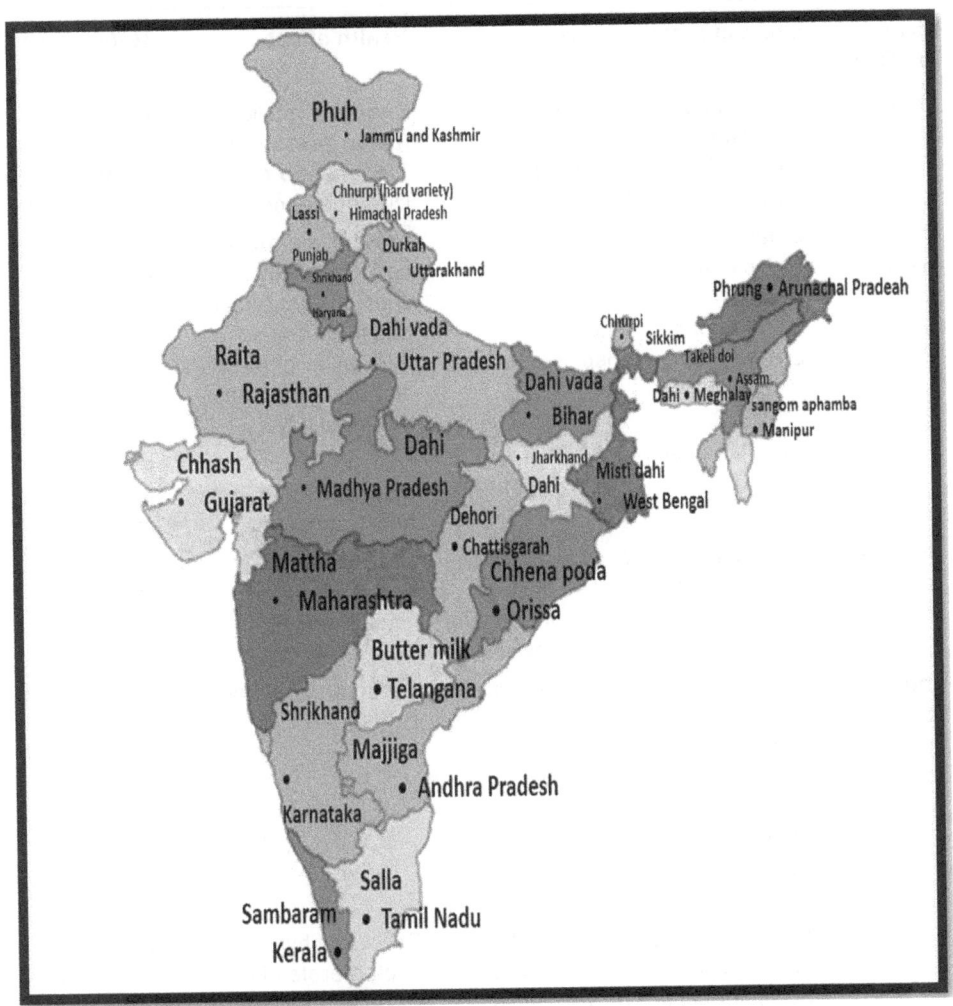

Fig. 1. Fermented milk products popular in different states of India

Different Traditional Fermented Milk Foods and their Bio-Functional Attributes

India is a place where plethora of fermented milk foods are available across different states since ancient times. The Indian traditional fermented milk products and their bio-functional attributes are summarized in Table 1. Different traditional fermented milk foods found in different states of India are discussed below

Table 1. Different traditional fermented milk products of India and their health benefits

Dairy Products	Characterized strains	Health effect	References
Shrikhand	*L. lactis* subsp. *diacetylactis*, *Leuconostoc* spp., *L. lactis* subsp. *lactis*, *Lb. delbrueckii* subsp. *bulgaricus* and *S. thermophilus*	Reduce systolic BP (blood pressure), Treat gastro enteritis, Diarrhoea and Acidity	(Srinivas *et al.*, 2017; Tamang *et al.*, 2016)
Kalari / Kradi	*L. lactis* subsp. *diacytylactis*, *L. lactis* subsp. *cremoris*, *L. lactis* subsp. *lactis*, *S. thermophilus* and *Lb. delbruekii* subsp. *bulgaricus*	Prevent diarrhoea, cancers, Reduce cholesterol concentration in blood, Alleviation of intestinal disorders and raises the immunity	(Caggia *et al.*, 2015; Punoo *et al.*, 2018)
Buttermilk	No such bacterial strain in use	Cure cardiovascular disease, Inflammation and Cancer	(Contarini and Povolo, 2013)
Misti Dahi	*Lb. acidophilus*, *L. lactis* subsp. *lactis*, *Lb. delbrueckii* subsp. *bulgaricus*, *S. sabbblivarius* subsp. *thermophilus* and *S. cerevisiae*	Cure various gastrointestinal diseases	(Adak *et al.*, 2013; Tamang *et al.*, 2020)
Churpi/ Churapi/ Durkah	*L. lactis*, *Lb. helveticus*, *A. syzygii*, *A. lovaniensis*, *A. pasteurianus*, *L. mesenteroides*, *S. cohnii*, *G. oxydans*, *Lb. delbrueckii*, *L. pseudomesenteroides*, *P. fluorescens*, *L. raffinolactis*, *A. tropicalis*, *Lb. gasseri* and *L. Brevis*	Cure cancer, Lowers Cholesterol	(Shangpliang *et al.*, 2018; Ghatani and Tamang, 2017)
Dahi	*L. lactis*, *S. lactis*, *S. diacetylactis*, *Leuconostoc* spp., *S. cremoris*, *Lb. bulgaricus*, *Lb. acidophilus*, *Lb. casei* and *S. thermophilus*	Decrease hypercholesterolemia, Cure abdominal discomfort, Diarrhoea, Cramps, Flatulence and Nausea	(Mudgal *et al.*, 2017)

[Table Contd.

Contd. Table]

Dairy Products	Characterized strains	Health effect	References
Lassi	*Lb. acidophilus, L. lactis* subsp. *lactis, L. lactis* subsp. *cremoris, L. lactis* subsp. *diacetylactis, S. thermophilus, Lb. bulgaricus*	Cure various gastrointestinal disorders like diarrhoea, Dysentery, Stomach bloating, Nausea and Vomiting	(Padghan *et al.*, 2015; Tamang *et al.*, 2016)
Phuh	Not reported	Exhibitantioxidative, Anti-hypertensive, Antimicrobial, Immunomodulatory and Opioid or mineral-carrying activity	(Korhonen and Pihlanto, 2007)
Azaco Cheese	Not reported	Exhibitantioxidative, Anti-hypertensive, Antimicrobial, Immunomodulatory and Opioid or mineral-carrying activity	(Korhonen and Pihlanto, 2007)
Somar	*Lb. paracasei* subsp. *pseudoplantarum* and *L. lactis* subsp. *cremoris*	Cures digestive disorder, Diarrhoea	(Dewan and Tamang, 2007)
Mattha	*Lb. acidophilus, Lb. sporogenes,* and *Lb. rhamnosus*	Similar like butter milk	(Tamang *et al.*, 2020)
Rabadi	*Micrococcus spp., Bacillus spp., P. acidilactici, S. lactis* and *S. cremoris*	Reduce coronary heart disease, Cancer, Maintain blood glucose level	(Tamang *et al.*, 2020)
Chhu	*Lb. farciminis, Lb. brevis, Lb. alimentarius, Lb. salivarius, L. lactis* subsp. *Cremoris*	Exhibit possible probiotic characteristic	(Dewan and Tamang, 2006)
Chilka	*Lactobacillus spp., Lactococcus spp., Leuconostoc spp.* and *Streptococcus spp.*	Anti-fungal activity	(Adak *et al.*, 2013)
Bandel Cheese	Not reported	Not reported	(Tamang *et al.*, 2020)

1. **Shrikhand:** Shrikhand is a semi soft, sweet and sour, healthy desert, fermented milk product prepared from buffalo milk. It is very popular in western part of India (Kumar *et al.*, 2011). *Lactococcus lactis* subsp. *diacetylactis, Leuconostoc* spp. and *Lactococcus lactis* subsp. *lactis*. have been used in equal ratio during production of Shrikhand. Various probiotic cultures like *Lactobacillus delbrueckii* subsp. *bulgaricus* and *Streptococcus thermophilus* have also been used. Shrikhand can reduce systolic BP (blood pressure) in hypertensive patient. Some studies mentioned that intake of shrikhand improves human immune system. The enhancement of conjugated linoleic acid (0.5-1.0%) during manufacturing shows anticarcinogenic activity (Sarkar, 2008). Shrikhand was also recommended to treat many diseases like gastro enteritis, diarrhoea and acidity (Srinivas *et al.*, 2017). These health beneficial attributes help to make Shrikhand a potential fermented food for combating several infectious diseases.

2. **Kalari or Kradi:** Kalari is a popular ripened cheese of Jammu, prepared from buffalo milk acidified with buttermilk or cultured skimmed milk (Punoo *et al.*, 2018; Mushtaq *et al.*, 2019). It has high moisture content, sour aroma and smooth texture and bright appearance. The chief microbiota of kalari cheese are aerobic *psychrotrophs, lactococci, thermophilic* and mesophilic *lactobacilli,* mesophilic aerobes and *Enterobacteriaceae* (Mushtaq *et al.*, 2015). Kalari exhibits health benefits due to itsantioxidative property (Mushtaq *et al.*, 2015). Kalari cheese containing probiotic strains like *Lactobacill* and *Bifidobacterium* exhibit greater antioxidant activity (Caggia *et al.*, 2015). Mushtaq *et al.* (2018) reported that the use of pomegranate peel extract incorporated zein film exhibit antioxidative and antimicrobial properties in kalari cheese. Kalari/Kradi has the potential to attract numerous scope of research due to very limited available resources on its biofunctional properties.

3. **Buttermilk / Chhash:** Buttermilk/ Chhash is mainly prepared as a by-product during manufacturing of butter. It is highly refreshing drink with a thin consistency and regarded as one of the most popular fermented milk product, found in all over India. Buttermilk is also called as Khachu in Bhutan and Mohi in Nepal. It is rich in milk fat globule membrane (MFGM), especially phospholipids and sphingolipids (Crespo *et al.*, 2018). The MFGM leads to exhibit various bio-functional attributes like cholesterol-lowering, anti-inflammatory, chemotherapeutic, ACE inhibitory properties and anti-neurodegenerative effects (Conway *et al.*, 2014). The sphingolipids in buttermilk are capable of preventing occurrence of colon cancer whereas phospholipids exhibit antimicrobial activity (Conway *et al.*, 2014). It is also beneficial to treat cardiovascular disease, inflammation and cancer (Contarini

and Povolo, 2013). Buttermilk is also popular for its therapeutic and functional properties which helpin enhancing human immunity (Nirgude *et al.*, 2013). Buttermilk solids favour the growth of several probiotics which are highly essential for gut microbiota (Mudgil and Barak, 2019). Butter milk has been used to cure the gastrointestinal disorder since ancient time (Mudgal *et al.*, 2017). Buttermilk may be a good source of immunity boosting components if taken regularly.

4. **Misti Dahi:** Misti dahi is a delicious traditional Indian fermented milk product popular mainly in West Bengal. It has creamy light brown appearance, smooth body with firm texture, slight acidic taste with pleasant aroma (Kumar *et al.*, 2018). Lactic acid bacteria such as *Lb. acidophilus, L. lactis subsp. lactis, Lb. delbrueckii subsp. bulgaricus, Streptococcus salivarius subs. thermophilus and S. cerevisiae* have been used for misti dahi preparation. They exhibit potential bio-functional properties. Misti dahi also helps to cure various gastro-intestinal diseases (Tamang, 2020). It has the potential to exhibit antimicrobial and antioxidant activities (Tamang, 2020). Probiotic cultures containing *Lb. helveticus* and *S. thermophillus* have been isolated from misti dahi (Saikia and Mishra, 2017) which are proved to be effective to cure gastro-intestinal disorders of consumers. More researches are required to explore the health benefits of Misti dahi and their role in immunity boosting.

5. **Chhurpi/ Churapi/Durkah:** Chhurpi is an uncommon variety of cheese, prepared from yak milk and mostly found in Himalayan regions of India. A traditional fermentation technique known as back-slopping has been applied for preparation of chhurpi. This technique has greater potential to produce antimicrobials such as bacteriocins

   Three varieties of chhurpi are namely hard chhurpi, soft chhurpi and dudh chhurpi are generally found in market. It is similar to cottage cheese with rubbery texture and sour taste. The fresh chhurpi has excellent flavour.

   Huge diversifications of bacterial strains are observed in chhurpi which make the product unique from other fermented milk foods. The isolated strains include *L. lactis, Lb. helveticus, A. syzygii, A. lovaniensis, A. pasteurianus, L. mesenteroides, S. cohnii, G. oxydans, Lb. delbrueckii, L. pseudomesenteroides, P. fluorescens, L. raffinolactis, A. tropicalis and Lb. gasseri* (Shangpliang *et al.*, 2018). These all strains have the potential to exhibit bio-functional properties like antimicrobial, antioxidative, cholesterol lowering, immunomodulatory, ACE inhibitory, anti-inflammatory, anti-carcinogenic, anti-diabetic, and anti-allergenic properties related to our immune system.

6. **Dahi:** Dahi is a traditional fermented milk product prepared from boiled cow milk or buffalo milk followed by cooling and addition of suitable culture. It is the most popular fermented dairy product found all over the India. Dahi also poses biofunctional properties due to formation of peptides during fermentation. The most common microorganisms found in traditional dahi are *L. lactis, S. lactis, S. diacetylactis, Leuconostoc sp., S. cremoris, Lactobacillus bulgaricus, Lactobacillus acidophilus, Lactobacillus casei* and *Streptococcus thermophilus.* Dahi exhibit bio-functional characteristics due to the probiotic nature of the microorganisms present in it. Dahi is a rich source of essential nutrients. It contains thiamine, riboflavin, folic acid, niacin, and cyanocobalamin. It is also a source of essential minerals like calcium, potassium, phosphorus, magnesium, sodium required for immunity boosting. Probiotic cultures like *L. acidophilus* and *B. bifidum* along with normal dahi culture (*L. lactis* subsp. *cremoris* and *L. lactis* subsp. *diacetylactis*) exhibit anticarcinogenic activity (Rajpal and Kansal, 2008). Dahi prepared with strains of *L. acidophilus* and *B. bifidum* culture show anti-oxidative property (Rajpal and Kansal, 2009). Dahi also exhibits anti-diabetic activity by suppressing streptozotocin induced diabetes and restrict depletion of insulin (Yadav *et al.*, 2008). Dahi also decreases hypercholesterolemia and reduce atherogenic index by increasing high-density lipoprotein (HDL) (Mudgal *et al.*, 2017).

Starter cultures used in dahi are location specific. Different non- descriptive starter cultures are found in traditionally prepared Indian dahi which may have potential health benefits. More systematic study is required to explore the full potential of health benefits exerted by dahi.

7. **Lassi:** Lassi is a refreshing drink prepared from heat treated milk with addition of sugar and suitable culture. Sometimes various food additives are used to enhance it's therapeutic and nutritional properties as well as its acceptability. Lassi is a high energetic drink due to its high nutritional qualities. It is a rich source of amino acids, peptides, vitamins, minerals, etc. It contains low amount of fat which is acceptable for obese people. High amount of calcium content helps to improve bone health. Lassi contains higher amount of vitamin D which helps to build up strong immune system. Lassi is a good source of lactic acid bacteria which help to improve the digestion system. It helps to cure various gastrointestinal disorders like diarrhoea, dysentery, stomach bloating, nausea and vomiting (Padghan *et al.*, 2015; Tamang *et al.*, 2016). Lassi containing probiotic culture *L. acidophilus* exhibits antioxidative and ACE inhibitory properties (Padghan *et al.*, 2017). Biofunctional properties of lassi are mainly attributed to the peptides present in it. Full potential of lassi as an immunity boosting fermented beverage is yet to be explored.

8. **Other fermented milk products:** Numerous lesser known traditional fermented milk products are available across India which may exhibit biofunctional properties (Table 1). Phuh or Azaco cheese is an acid coagulated soft cheese made from colostrum milk fermented with mesophilic starter culture which is found in Jammu and Kashmir. Sherpas of high hill use to take Somar which is an endemic fermented dairy product prepared from yak milk or cow milk. It cures digestive disorder and helps to raise the appetite (Tamang, 2020). Mattha is a similar product like buttermilk in which roasted cumin, ginger, green chillies and curry leaves are added. Rabadi is a cereal based fermented milk products prepared from buttermilk, popular in North- western part of India. Chhu is a strong flavoured cheese prepared from yalk milk exhibit potential antagonism properties, found in sikkim. People of Chilika (Odisha) prepared fermented milk in bamboo basket, especially from buffalo milk. Bandel cheese is a fermented dairy product popular in Bandel of West Bengal, carrying significant amount of lactic acid bacteria. No scientific study has been reported so far on these products. Scientific intervention is needed to discover the biofunctional attributes of these product for exploring potential health benefits.

CONCLUSION

Fermented milk products are popular throughout the world due to their nutritional qualities and health benefits. Bio-functional properties of fermented products are observed as a result of fermentation caused by the microorganisms present in it. India boasts numerous traditional fermented milk products most of which are not commonly known to us. These products also come up with unknown bio-functional properties which need to be recorded. In this present pandemic situation, these products can help to boost up our immune system to combat with covid-19 virus. This study welcomes possible researches to be done on these products and their possible bio-functional attributes.

REFERENCES

Adak A, Parua S, Maity C, Ghosh K, Halder SK, Das Mohapatra PK, Mondal KC (2013) A comparative study of its physico-chemical parameters with other marketed curds. *Indian J Exp Biol* **51**: 910–918

Caggia C, De Angelis M, Pitino I, Pino A, Randazzo CL (2015) Probiotic features of Lactobacillus strains isolated from Ragusano and Pecorino Siciliano cheeses. *Food Microbiol* **50**:109-17.

Chakrabarti S, Guha S, Majumder K (2018) Food-derived bioactive peptides in human health: Challenges and opportunities. *Nutri* **10(11):** 1738.

Contarini G, Povolo M (2013) Phospholipids in milk fat: composition, biological and technological significance, and analytical strategies. *Int J Mol Sci* **14(2):** 2808-31.

Conway V, Gauthier SF, Pouliot Y (2014) Buttermilk: much more than a source of milk phospholipids. *Anim Fron* **4(2):** 44-51.

Crespo MC, Tomé-Carneiro J, Gómez-Coronado D, Burgos-Ramos E, García-Serrano A *et al.* (2018) Modulation of miRNA expression in aged rat hippocampus by buttermilk and krill oil. *Scientific reports* **8(1):** 1-2.

Dewan S, Tamang JP (2006) Microbial and analytical characterization of Chhu-A traditional fermented milk product of the Sikkim Himalayas. *J Sci Ind Res* **65:** 747-752.

Dewan S, Tamang JP (2007) Dominant lactic acid bacteria and their technological properties isolated from the Himalayan ethnic fermented milk products. *Antonie van Leeuwenhoek* **92(3):** 343-52.

Ghatani K, Tamang B (2017) Assessment of probiotic characteristics of lactic acid bacteria isolated from fermented yak milk products of Sikkim, India: Chhurpi, Shyow, and Khachu. *Food Biotechnol* **31(3):** 210-32.

Gortzi O, Tsakali E, Chatzilazarou A, Galidi A, Houhoula D, Tsaknis J, Sflomos C (2015) E-food science project: bio-functional foods. **In:** Proceedings of the 2nd International Conference on Food and Biosystems Engineering, Mykonos Island, Greece, pp. 119-126.

Haque E, Chand R, Kapila S (2008) Biofunctional properties of bioactive peptides of milk origin. *Food Rev Int* **25(1):** 28-43.

Hati S, Mishra BK (2015) Health benefits of milk derived biofunctional peptides–A review *Int J Bio-Res Env Agri Sci* **1(2):** 14-20.

Korhonen H, Pihlanto A (2007) Technological options for the production of health-promoting proteins and peptides derived from milk and colostrum. *Curr Pharm Des* **13(8):** 829-43.

Kumar S, Bhat ZF, Kumar P (2011) Effect of apple pulp and Celosia argentea on the quality characteristics of Shrikhand. *Am J Food Technol* **6(9):**1-8.

Kumar S, Rasane P, Nimmanapalli R (2018) Optimisation of a process for production of pomegranate pulp and flaxseed powder fortified probiotic Greek dahi. *Int J Dairy Technol* **71(3):** 753-63.

Linares DM, Gomez C, Renes E, Fresno JM, Tornadijo ME, Ross RP, Stanton C (2017) Lactic acid bacteria and bifidobacteria with potential to design natural biofunctional health-promoting dairy foods. *Front Microbiol* **8:**846.

Mohanty DP, Mohapatra S, Misra S, Sahu PS (2016) Milk derived bioactive peptides and their impact on human health–A review. *Saudi J Bio Sci* **23(5):** 577-83.

Mudgal SP, Prajapati JB (2017) Dahi—An Indian Naturally Fermented Yogurt. **In:** Yogurt in Health and Disease Prevention. Nagendra P. Shah (ed), Elsevier, London, pp. 353-369.

Mudgil D, Barak S (2019) Dairy-Based Functional Beverages. **In:** Milk-Based Beverages. Alexandru M.G &alina M.H (ed), Elsevier, Duxford, pp. 67-93.

Mushtaq M, Gani A, Gani A, Punoo HA, Masoodi FA (2018) Use of pomegranate peel extract incorporated zein film with improved properties for prolonged shelf life of fresh Himalayan cheese (Kalari/kradi). *Innov Food Sci Emerg Technol* **48:** 25-32.

Mushtaq M, Gani A, Masoodi FA (2019) Himalayan cheese (Kalari/Kradi) fermented with different probiotic strains: In vitro investigation of nutraceutical properties. *LWT-Food Science Technol* **104:** 53-60.

Mushtaq M, Gani A, Shetty PH, Masoodi FA, Ahmad M (2015) Himalayan cheese (Kalari/kradi): Effect of different storage temperatures on its physicochemical, microbiological and antioxidant properties. *LWT-Food Science Technol* **63(2):** 837-45.

Nanda DK, Singh R, Tomar SK, Dash SK, Jayakumar S, Arora DK, Chaudhary R, Kumar D (2013) Indian Chilika curd–A potential dairy product for Geographical Indication registration. *Indian J Tradi Know* **12(4):** 707-713.

Nirgude R, Binorkar SV, Parlikar GR, Kirte MC, Savant DP (2013) Therapeutic and nutritional values of takra (buttermilk). *Int Res J Pharm* **4(2):** 29-31.

Padghan PV, Mann B, Sharma R, Bajaj R, Saini P (2017) Production of angiotensin-I-converting-enzyme-inhibitory peptides in fermented milks (Lassi) fermented by *Lactobacillus acidophillus* with consideration of incubation period and simmering treatment. *Int J Pept Res Ther* **23(1):** 69-79.

Padghan PV, Mann B, Sharma R, Kumar A (2015) Studies on bio-functional activity of traditional Lassi. *Indian J Tradi Know* **1(1):** 124-131.

Pophaly SD, Chauhan M, Lule V, Sarang P, Tarak J, Thakur K, Tomar SK (2018) Functional Starter Cultures for Fermented Dairy Products. **In:** Microbial Cultures and Enzymes in Dairy Technology IGI Global, pp. 54-68.

Punoo HA, Patil GR, Bijoy RR (2018) Textural and microstructural properties of Kradi cheese (an indigenous cheese of Jammu and Kashmir, India). *Int J Dairy Technol* **(2):** 372-81.

Rajpal S, Kansal VK (2008) Buffalo milk probiotic Dahi containing Lactobacillus acidophilus, Bifidobacteriumbifidum and Lactococcuslactis reduces gastrointestinal cancer induced by dimethylhydrazinedihydrochloride in rats. *Milchwissenschaft- Milk Sci Int J* **63(2):** 122-5.

Rajpal S, Kansal VK (2009) Probiotic Dahi containing Lactobacillus acidophilus and Bifidobacteriumbifidum stimulates immune system in mice. *Milchwissenschaft- Milk Sci Int J* **64(3):** 290-290.

Saikia G, Mishra BK (2017) Growth of Lactic Acid Bacteria in Milk for the Preparation of Functional Frozen Misti Dahi (Sweet Curd). *Int J Sci Res Sci Technol* **3(8):** 22-26.

Sarkar S (2008) Innovations in Indian fermented milk products: A review. *Food Biotechnol* **22:** 78-97.

Shangpliang HN, Rai R, Keisam S, Jeyaram K, Tamang JP (2018) Bacterial community in naturally fermented milk products of Arunachal Pradesh and Sikkim of India analysed by high-throughput amplicon sequencing. *Scientific Reports* **8(1):** 1532.

Srinivas J, Suneetha J, Maheswari KU, Kumari BA, Devi SS, Krishnaiah N (2017) Nutritional analysis of value added Shrikhand. *Int J Pharmacogn Phytochem* **6(5):** 1438-41.

Tamang JP (2020) Ethnic Fermented Foods and Beverages of India: Science History and Culture. Springer Nature.

Tamang JP, Shin DH, Jung SJ, Chae SW (2016) Functional properties of microorganisms in fermented foods. *Front Microbiol* **7:** 578.

Yadav H, Jain S, Sinha PR (2008) Oral administration of dahi containing probiotic Lactobacillus acidophilus and Lactobacillus casei delayed the progression of streptozotocin-induced diabetes in rats. *J Dairy Res* **75(2):** 189.

Immunity Boosting Functional Foods to Combat COVID-19, Pages: 189–196
Edited by: Apurba Giri
Copyright © 2021, Narendra Publishing House, Delhi, India

CHAPTER - 16

IMMUNE-BOOSTING ROLE OF ZINC AGAINST COVID-19

Abhinandan Rana

Assistant Professor
Dept. of Chemistry, Garhbeta College, Garhbeta, Paschim Medinipur-721 127, India
E-mail: ranaabhinandan@gmail.com

ABSTRACT

COVID-19 is a significant threat to healthcare worldwide. To combat against the coronavirus it is necessary to boost immunity in our body. For this purpose we have to take balanced diet regularly. Zinc is an essential trace element, involved in numerous biological processes including immunity. But we have seen that various developing countries suffering from serious zinc deficiency. Insufficiency of vitamins and minerals among vulnerable populations has increased the morbidity and risk of mortality. Zn deficiency causes immune dysfunction and numerous diseases. Zinc supplement may counter such deficiency. Therefore, zinc is a vital mineral at this COVID-19 pandemic situation as it has both anti-viral and immunomodulatory properties.

Keywords: Zinc, Covid-19, Immunity, Antioxidant

INTRODUCTION

Coronavirus disease (COVID-19) is a global public health concern caused by the novel coronavirus SARS-CoV-2 and represents a significant threat to healthcare worldwide. At first it was diagnosed on 31st December 2019, in Wuhan city, China. Then it was named as 2019 nCoV. After that World Health Organization (WHO) recalled it as COVID-19. This killing virus can easily be transferred from one person to another person via respiratory droplets and direct contact. The general symptoms of coronavirus infection are sore throat, cough, fever, body and muscle aches, loss of smell and taste and even diarrhea in some cases (Veverka *et al.*, 2009). For the treatment of COVID-19 patients the proper medicines are not discovered till now. Only various preventive measures like social distancing, wearing facial masks, hand gloves, frequently washing hands using soap or alcohol based hand sanitizers are advised to take people to reduce COVID-19 infection. Besides, different immunity boosting foods like vitamin C, vitamin D, vitamin A, Zinc, Selenium, Magnesium, garlic, ginger, turmeric etc are required in human body to combat against COVID-19. The trace elements are necessary in our body for the proper growth, development, physiology of the organism and immune function. Zinc is such kind of element after iron. As it cannot be stored in our body, we have to be taken up via food daily.

Recent studies have mentioned that in COVID-19 patients dietary supplementation could play a helpful role (Razzaque, 2020). Zinc is an important trace element and a strong antioxidant. The active site of about 300 enzymes (Prasad, 2003; Plum *et al.*, 2010; Osredkar and Sustar, 2011) contain zinc ion. Zn is especially crucial for human body because it acts in metabolism of carbohydrates, proteins and lipids (Prasad, 2017). Also it is important for cell growth and cell division, DNA and protein synthesis (Burjonrappa and Miller, 2012).

Insufficient dietary intake causes Zn deficiency in individuals. About 2 bn people in development country are suffering from Zn deficiency worldwide (Prasad, 2003). Micronutrients (vitamins and minerals) deficiencies are mainly observed in elderly people, COVID-19 patients, which increase the morbidity and risk of mortality (Grant *et al.*, 2020). As a result of zinc deficiency, the immune system of our body is deactivated and causes several diseases e.g., weight loss, hair loss, taste loss, delayed wounds healing, delayed sexual maturation, pneumonia, diarrhea, etc (Maretm and Sandstead, 2006). Zn supplementation and food fortification together play an important role to overcome these difficulties (Sanstead *et al.*, 2000; Lassi *et al.*, 2010). The functions of zinc in immunity to combat COVID-19 are discussed in this paper.

Zinc and COVID 19

As an essential micronutrient, the transition metal zinc is generally used for biological processes include normal growth, development, repair, metabolism, and maintenance of cell integrity and functionality (Prasad, 2013). In this COVID 19 pandemic situation, we may use zinc as a possible supportive treatment against coronavirus infection because of its antiviral as well as immune modulatory effect (Zhang and Liu, 2020; Skalny *et al.*, 2020).

Zinc has capable to generate CD4+ and CD8+ T cells. Furthermore, the number of T cells and NK cells is increased by zinc supplementation and it also helps to enhance IL-2. Besides, zinc strongly inhibits the viral replication and transcription complex of coronavirus (Velthuis *et al.*, 2010; Skalny *et al.*, 2020). It is mentioned that zinc supplementation may be utilized for the treatment of COVID-19 patients (Rahman and Idid, 2020). Different Studies have shown that zinc supplementation is able to decrease COVID-19 related symptoms such as lower respiratory tract infection (Finzi, 2020).

Zinc and Immunity

Zinc is very helpful nutrient for our immune system (Overbeck *et al.*, 2008; Prasad, 2008). It is necessary for normal development, cell division and cell activation, DNA synthesis, RNA transcription and natural killer (NK) cells. So due to lack of zinc, not only the production and functions of cytokines (messengers of the immune system) (Prasad, 2013) are disrupted but also the function of T and B cells, Phagocytosis, Macrophages, intracellular killing are all greatly affected.

There are two types of immunity systems, one is the innate immunity and the other is adaptive immunity (Turvey and Broide, 2010). In case of innate immunity system, at first polymorphonuclear cells (PMNs) reach to the site of infection and actively participate to recognition and elimination of the pathogens which enter into our body. They immediately catch pathogens by phagocytosis and destroy them through the invention of reactive oxygen species (ROS) (Haase and Rink, 2014). Macrophages and NK cells may also act the same.

The adaptive immunity system is controlled by extremely specific cells, the B and T lymphocytes. B lymphocytes play an important role in producing the antibodies particularly against an antigen, whereas T-lymphocytes act with the help of other immune cells and produced toxic particles in cytotoxic T lymphocytes. These two immunity systems are interlinked by the Dendritic cells (DCs) (Maywald *et al.*, 2017).

Mechanism of Zinc Effects

Figure 1 explains the effect of zinc on immune cells (Prasad, 2007). Zinc is an important constituent of thymulin, a thymic hormone engaged in maturation and separation of T-cells. Zinc dependent Th1 cytokines are IL-2 and IFN-γ. IL-2 is associated with the function of NK and T cytolytic cells. Macrophages-monocytes produce IL-12, which is also a zinc-dependent cytokine. Now macrophages-monocytes kill viruses, bacteria and parasites with the help of both IL-12 and

IFN-γ. Generally, zinc deficiency can't influence Th2 cytokines except IL-10, which is enhanced in the zinc deficient elderly human beings. Zinc supplementation removes this problem. Furthermore, increased IL-10 affects adversely Th1 and macrophage functions.

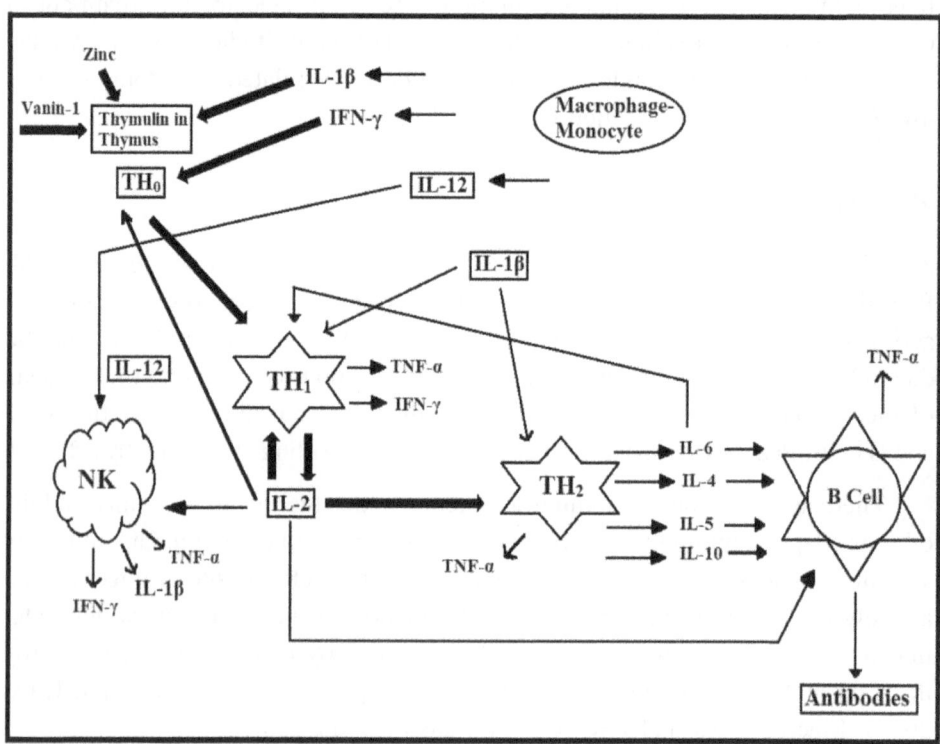

Fig. 1: Effect of Zinc on immune cells

Figure 2 demonstrates the function of zinc as an antioxidant and anti-inflammatory agent (Prasad, 2008; Prasad, 2009). NF-κB is activated by ROS. But the production of ROS is decreased by zinc. Zinc and SOD together resist NADPH oxidase. SOD (super oxide dismutase) is an enzyme, composed of two metals copper and zinc. It reduces the oxidative stress in the body. Metallothionein (MT) has 26 moles of cysteine per mole of protein and it is activated by zinc. The activation of NF-κB is inhibited by Zinc via A20. As a result the production of inflammatory cytokines and adhesion molecules is diminished. From the figure 2 it is also observed that zinc may have a precautionary role in cancer disease like colon cancer, prostate cancer, etc and in atherosclerosis.

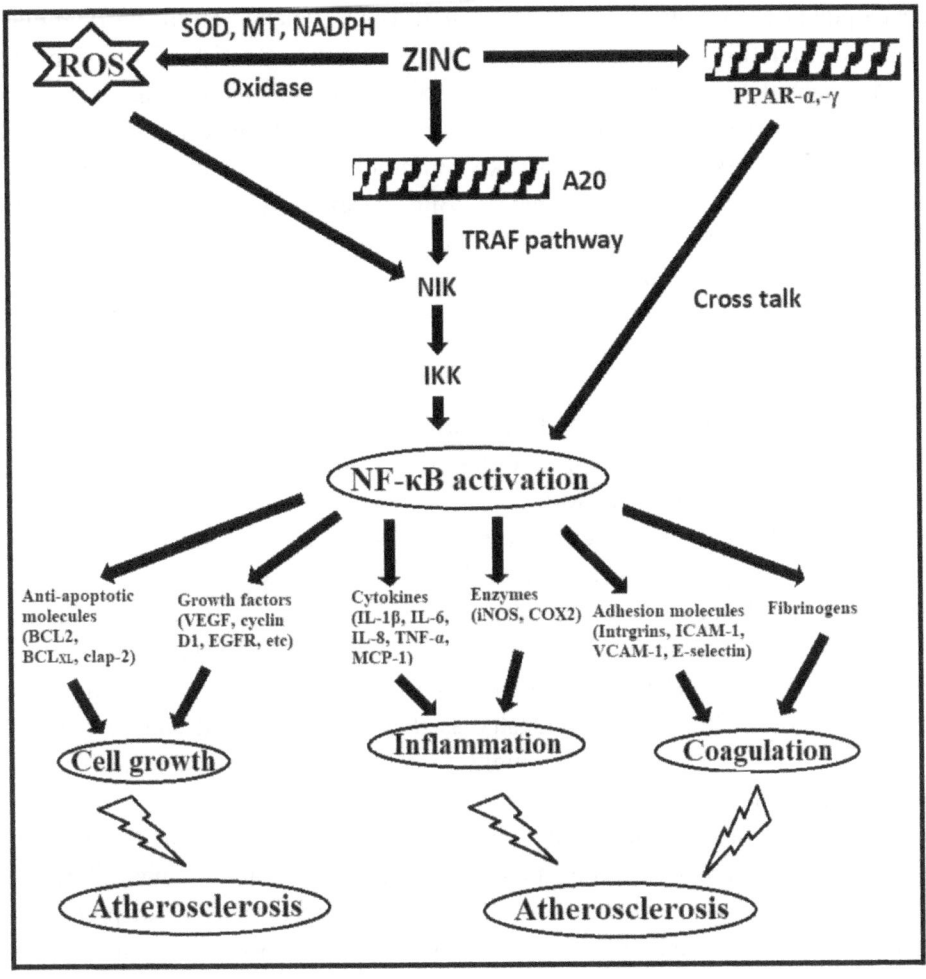

Fig. 2: Activity of zinc as an antioxidant and anti-inflammatory agent

Zinc Riched Foods

Zinc is an essential nutrient that acts a crucial role in immune system response, wound healing, synthesizing proteins and DNA, and many other bodily functions. The well-known recommended daily amount (RDA) of Zn for male and female are 11 mg and 8 mg respectively (Al-Fartusie and Mohssan, 2017). Zinc is found in various foods e.g., oysters, seafood (crab, lobster), nuts, seeds, shellfish, beans, chickpeas, fortified cereals, wheat, brown rice, oats, lentils, soybeans, dried peas, black-eyed peas, walnuts, peanuts, brazil nuts, red meat, poultry and yogurt. Besides almost all health supplements or multivitamins available in the market have zinc as oxide, sulfate, or citrate. Zinc containing foods are very much helpful to boost our immune system (Hemila et al., 2016). Consequently for the development of immune cell zinc is required. But deficiency of this nutrient may results dysfunction of our immune system and enhances the risk of infection and disease, including pneumonia. About 2 bn people are affected by zinc deficiency worldwide, among them older peoples are very common. However, it is mentioned that the respiratory tract infections like common cold (Science *et al.*, 2012) are greatly inhibited by zinc supplements. But the excessive intake of zinc may obstruct the absorption of copper in our body, which leads to increase the risk of infection (Dardenne, 2002).

Zinc Fortified Foods

Zinc fortified foods are extremely important nowadays as there are a limited natural sources of this nutrient. Peoples of various development countries are gradually habituated to use the fortified foods as heath supplement. Zinc deficiency among the vulnerable people can also be reduced by this way. Recently five zinc compounds are used for fortification. These are zinc oxide, zinc sulfate, zinc chloride, zinc gluconate and zinc stearate (Rosado, 2003). These compounds are also enlisted by the US Food and Drug Administration named as GRAS (generally recognized as safe) (Hess and Brown, 2009). Zinc oxide and zinc sulfate are generally utilized by the food industry as they are low-priced among the five compounds. Zinc fortification was highly initiated in China and Mexico (Das *et al.*, 2013a). Bhutta et al. reported that serum zinc concentration is increased markedly by both milk- and cereal-based products (Das *et al.*, 2013b). Besides zinc-fortified various milk products are useful for infants and young children to improve the zinc status in their body. Also to develop the growth of premature baby and malnourished children these milk products have been widely used (Hess and Brown, 2009).

CONCLUSION

Vitamins and minerals (micronutrients) are necessary for metabolism, growth and other functions of the human body. Zinc is a trace element that is required for the development of immune cells, DNA synthesis and cell propagation. Zinc may be used for the treatment of COVID-19 patients due to its dual anti-viral and immune modulatory properties. As there is no such appropriate treatment discovered till now, so we have to take healthy diet regularly to develop immunity in our body to combat against coronavirus. With the aids of health supplementation and fortification of foods, deficiency of vitamins and minerals may be overcome. Lastly, good food habits are incredibly helpful to boost our immune system.

REFERENCES

Al-Fartusie FS, Mohssan SN (2017) Essential Trace Elements and Their Vital Roles in Human Body. *Indian J Adv Chem Sci* **5(3):** 127-136.

Burjonrappa SC, Miller M (2012) Role of trace elements in parenteral nutrition support of the surgical neonate. *J Pediatr Surg* **47:** 760-771.

Dardenne M (2002) Zinc and immune function. *Eur J Clin Nutr* **56:** S20-S23.

Das JK, Kumar R, Salam RA, Bhutta ZA (2013a) Systematic Review of Zinc Fortification Trials. *Ann Nutr Metab* **62:** 44-56.

Das JK, Kumar R, Salam RA, Bhutta ZA (2013b) Micronutrient fortification of food and its impact on woman and child health: a systematic review. *Syst Rev* **2:** 67-90.

Finzi E (2020) Treatment of SARS-CoV-2 with high dose oral zinc salts: a report on four patients. *Int J Infect Dis* **99:** 307-309.

Grant WB, Lahore H, McDonnell SL, Baggerly CA, French CB, Aliano JL, Bhattoa HP (2020) Evidence that vitamin D supplementation could reduce risk of influenza and COVID-19 infections and deaths. *Nutrients* **12 (4):** 988-1006.

Haase H, Rink L (2014) Zinc signals and immune function. *Biofactors* **40:** 27-40.

Hemila H, Petrus EJ, Fitzgerald JT, Prasad A (2016) Zinc acetate lozenges for treating the common cold: an individual patient data meta-analysis. *Br J Clin Pharmacol* **82(5):** 1393-1398.

Hess SY, Brown KH (2009) Impact of zinc fortification on zinc nutrition. *Food Nutr Bull* **30:** S79-107.

Lassi ZS, Haider BA, Bhutta ZA (2010) Zinc supplementation for the prevention of pneumonia in children aged 2 months to 59 months. *Cochrane Database Syst Rev* **12:** CD005978.

Maretm W, Sandstead HH (2006) Zinc requirements and the risks and benefits of zinc supplementation. *J Trace Elem Med Biol* **20:** 3-18.

Maywald M, Wessels I, Rink L (2017) Zinc Signals and Immunity. *Int J Mol Sci* **18:** 2222-2255.

Osredkar J, Sustar N (2011) Copper and zinc, biological role and significance of copper/zinc imbalance. *J Clin Toxicol* **S3:** 1-18.

Overbeck S, Rink L, Haase H (2008) Modulating the immune response by oral zinc supplementation: a single approach for multiple diseases. *Arch Immunol Ther Exp* **56:** 15-30.

Plum L, Rink L, Haase H (2010) The essential toxin: Impact of zinc on human health. *Int J Environ Res Public Health* **7(4):** 1342-1365.

Prasad AS (2003) Zinc deficiency: Has been known of for 40 years but ignored by global health organizations. *Br Med J* **326(7386):** 409-410.

Prasad AS (2007) Zinc: mechanisms of host defense. *J Nutr* **137:** 1345-1349.

Prasad AS (2008) Clinical, immunological, anti-inflammatory and antioxidant roles of zinc. *Exp Gerontol* **43:** 370-377.

Prasad AS (2009) Zinc: role in immunity, oxidative stress and chronic inflammation. *Curr Opin Clin Nutr Metab Care* **12:** 646-652.

Prasad AS (2013) Discovery of human zinc deficiency: its impact on human health and disease. *Adv Nutr* **4:** 176-190.

Prasad AS (2017) Discovery of Zinc for Human Health and Biomarkers of Zinc Deficiency. **In:** Molecular, Genetic, and Nutritional Aspects of Major and Trace Minerals. Collins JF (ed). Academic Press, Cambridge, pp. 241 260.

Rahman MT, Idid SZ (2020) Can Zn Be a Critical Element in COVID-19 Treatment? *Biol Trace Elem Res* 1-9.

Razzaque MS (2020) COVID-19 Pandemic: Can Maintaining Optimal Zinc Balance Enhance Host Resistance? *Tohoku J Exp Med* **251(3):** 175-181.

Rosado JL (2003) Zinc and Copper: Proposed Fortification Levels and Recommended Zinc Compounds. *J Nutr* **133(9):** 2985S-2989S.

Sanstead HH, Frederickson CJ, Penland JG (2000) Zinc nutriture as related to brain. *J Nutr* **130:** 140S-146S.

Science M, Johnstone J, Roth DE, Guyatt G, Loeb M (2012) Zinc for the treatment of the common cold: A systematic review and meta-analysis of randomized controlled trials. *Can Med Assoc J* **184:** E551-E561.

Skalny AV, Rink L, Ajsuvakova OP, Aschner M, Gritsenko VA, Alekseenko SI, Svistunov AA, Petrakis D, Spandidos DA, Aaseth J (2020) Zinc and respiratory tract infections: perspectives for COVID 19. *Int J Mol Med* **46 (1):** 17–26.

Turvey SE, Broide DH (2010) Innate immunity. *J Allergy Clin Immunol* **125:** S24-32.

Velthuis AJT, Worm SHV, Sims AC, Baric RS, Snijder EJ, Hemert MJV (2010) Zn^{2+} inhibits coronavirus and arterivirus RNA polymerase activity in vitro and zinc ionophores block the replication of these viruses in cell culture. *PLoS Pathog* **6 (11):** e1001176.

Veverka DV, Wilson C, Martinez MA, Wenger R, Tamosuinas A (2009) Use of zinc supplements to reduce upper respiratory infections in United States Air Force Academy Cadets. *Complement Ther Clin Pract* **15:** 91-95.

Zhang L, Liu Y (2020) Potential interventions for novel coronavirus in China: A systematic review. *J Med Virol* **92:** 479 490.

Immunity Boosting Functional Foods to Combat COVID-19, Pages: 197–211
Edited by: Apurba Giri
Copyright © 2021, Narendra Publishing House, Delhi, India

CHAPTER - 17

VITAMIN D SUPPLEMENTATION TO COMBAT COVID-19: A REVIEW

Chaitali Bose

Ph.D Scholar, P.G. Dept. of Physiology, Hooghly Mohsin College,
Chinsurah, Hoogly-712101, West Bengal, India
E-mail: chaitali.bose85@gmail.com

ABSTRACT

Corona Virus Disease-2019 or COVID-19 is the ongoing global pandemic caused by SARS-COV-2 (Severe Acute Respiratory Syndrome Corona Virus 2) which affects mostly the respiratory system in humans, producing mild symptoms like fever, dry cough to severe life threatening complications like pneumonia, ARDS (Acute Respiratory Distress Syndrome) and others, ultimately leading to death. Elder population and people with different co morbidities like hypertension, diabetes, cardio vascular diseases or chronic kidney disease are more susceptible to get infected by this deadly virus. Amidst plenty of explored and unexplored risk factors which exacerbate COVID complications, reports from different European and other countries have identified poor serum concentration of vitamin D (25-hydroxy cholecalciferol <25nmol/L) is one of them. Vitamin D deficiency is found among elderly and black population; in home residents and even in various comorbidities. Besides its well defined role on musculo-skeletal system, vitamin D has prominent effects on host immune response, Renin-angiotensis-System (RAS) and many other extra-skeletal activities- which might serve the link between vitamin D deficiency and fatal outcome of COVID-19. Clinically it is proved that supplementation of this vitamin is beneficial to treat acute respiratory tract infection, tuberculosis, pneumonia or ARDS. Though the therapeutic effect of vitamin D supplementation in COVID-19 is still a subject of further investigations but when vitamin D deficiency is prevalent, then supplementation of vitamin D or consuming rich sources of vitamin D would likely to be beneficial for reducing the risk of the disease or its severity.

Keywords: COVID-19, Vitamin D, Immune-modulation, Renin-Angiotensin-System, Supplementation.

Background

Corona Virus Disease 2019 or COVID-19 pandemic is the biggest ever threat to mankind after the World War II. When an epidemiological transition has taken place across the world and percentage of global death and disabilities from Non-Communicable Diseases (NCDs) are increasing at a fast pace, then COVID-19, a highly contagious disease has emerged and claimed millions of lives worldwide. This disease was first identified as an outbreak with substantial cases of severe pneumonia of unknown reason in Wuhan city of Hubei province in central China and on 31st December 2019 Chinese health authority brought it under the scanner of World Health Organization (WHO). Later on 7th January of 2020, the causative agent was recognised from a patient's throat swab and this pathogen was named as novel corona virus (2019-nCOV) by WHO (Hui *et al.*, 2020; Wang *et al.*, 2020). It was again renamed as SARS COV-2 (severe acute respiratory distress corona virus 2) afterwards and the disease was named as COVID-19 (corona virus disease 2019). When there was increased number of fatality, confirmed and suspected cases of COVID-19 in China, then 18 other countries also reported confirmed cases of COVID-19 in the end of January. On 30th January, WHO has announced this disease as Public Health Emergency of International Concern (Harapan *et al.*, 2020; Singhal, 2020). But the frightening level of spread, magnitude and severity of this highly communicable disease has soon made WHO to characterize it as a pandemic on 11th March (WHO, 2020). As of 23rd August, 2020 the confirmed cases are 23,057,288 and 800,906 people died of it globally (covering 216 countries or territories) and in India the number of confirmed cases are over 3 million along with 56,706 deaths (WHO, 2020).

The Virus Behind

The virus, isolated and identified by the research team was a corona virus which is >95% genetically homologous with the corona virus of bat family and also has >70% homology with earlier prevailed SARS-COV (Singhal, 2020).

This virus belongs to coronaviridae family and coronavirinae subfamily. This subfamily contains four genera, namely alpha, beta, gamma and delta corona virus; among which alpha and beta corona virus can infect human. SARS-COV2 is a beta corona virus together with SARS-COV (Severe Acute Respiratory Syndrome Corona Virus) and MERS-COV (Middle East Respiratory Syndrome Corona Virus) which prevailed in 2002 and 2012 respectively and caused mild to severe respiratory distress (Burrell *et al.*, 2016; Unhale *et al.*, 2020).

Structurally this virus is a positive sense single stranded enveloped RNA virus. Though it is thought that bat is the primary host of this virus but intermediate host might play role to transmit this virus to human which needs further investigations (Li, 2015; Lu et al., 2020).

'Corona' is a *Latin* word which means 'crown', the spike proteins which protrude on the surface-envelop of the virus, give crown like structure. These spike proteins facilitate entry of this virus into human cell through binding to the target cell receptors (Richman et al., 2016).

Clinical Manifestations

Clinical manifestation of COVID-19 varies largely from subject to subject, which might results 'asymptomatic' state to mild or moderate symptoms or severe life-threatening complications. Common mild to moderate clinical features include sneezing, dry cough, chest pain, headache, fever, breathing trouble, fatigue or myalgia. Less common symptoms include gastro-intestinal disturbance like nausea or vomiting, abdominal pain and even acute diarrhoea may occur. Severe complications are hypoxemia, Acute Respiratory Distress Syndrome (ARDS), pneumonia, shock, arrhythmia, acute injuries to several organs like cardiac, lung or kidney injuries which might lead to multi organ failure and ultimately death (Chen et al., 2020; Huang et al., 2020; Unhale et al., 2020).

Risk Factors Associated with COVID-19

Elderly population, people with obesity and other co-morbidities like hypertension, insulin resistance, diabetes, cardio vascular disease, Chronic Obstructive Pulmonary Disease (COPD), cancer or chronic kidney problems are found to be suffered from the severity of the disease (Centers for Disease Control and Prevention, 2020)

Deficiency of Vitamin D as a Risk Factor

During this pandemic era, when researchers are either looking for protective dietary and therapeutic agents or investigating associated risk factors of COVID-19, vitamin D has emerged as an important agent in this context. Adequacy of serum vitamin D level has been thought to be protective therapeutic or dietary agent in one hand, whereas in other hand deficiency of vitamin D has found to be a risk factor for this disease (Trovas and Tournis, 2020).

According to the Endocrine Society Task Force when serum vitamin D level (25-OH-cholecalciferol) is <20 ng/ml is defined as vitamin D deficiency, 21-29 ng/ml is insufficient and >30 ng/ml is termed as sufficient (Holick *et al.*, 2011).

People with advanced ages, black population, obese people, persons on sedentary lifestyle, home residents, non ambulatory people and persons with different co-morbidities like hypertension, diabetes, cardiovascular disease, chronic kidney disease are often vitamin D deficient (Palacios and Gonzalez, 2014; Graedel *et al.*, 2016).

Now vitamin D deficiency has become a pandemic worldwide where more than one billion people are suffering from severe deficiency. Countries of northern latitude, poor exposure to sunlight, effect of drugs, poor diet, poor endogenous production and metabolism, seasonal variation, medical conditions pull down serum vitamin D level in people living even in tropical and subtropical countries (Palacios and Gonzalez, 2014; Biesalski, 2020). In India this deficiency also prevails ranging from 60%-90% of total population (Aparna *et al.*, 2018).

Literature Behind

Back in 1930, cod liver oil a rich source of vitamin D was used to treat common cold and associated acute upper respiratory tract infection among industrial employees (Martineau and Forouhi, 2020). Since then ample observational or experimental studies or clinical trials have been done which have unveiled a clear association between low circulating serum vitamin D and increased risks of common cold, flu, epidemic influenza, acute respiratory tract infection, epithelial damage, community-pneumonia, inflammation of alveolus or hypoxia and other viral infections. And many studies showed protective effect of supplementation of this vitamin against flu, common cold, influenza, tuberculosis, pulmonary lesions induced by advanced stages of tuberculosis, pneumonia, asthma, COPD or even ARDS (Dancer *et al.*, 2015; Quraishi *et al.*, 2015; Ali, 2020; Suvarna and Mohan, 2020; Verdoia and Luca, 2020). These clinical manifestations even in COVID-19 hypothesised its association with the disease.

Though data obtained on 20th May, 2020 from twenty European countries showed negative co-relation between mean vitamin D level and cases of COVID-19 or deaths due to it. But many other studies have opposed that finding and showed significant relationship behind low vitamin D and prevalence or severity of the disease. Through various retrospective observational studies in countries like UK, USA and Belgium or in many south Asian countries have divulged that elder people, obese or people with pre medical conditions with low vitamin D concentration is significantly associated with severity of COVID cases (Ali, 2020; Daneshkhah *et al.*, 2020; Hastie *et al.*, 2020). Study in USA by Li *et al.* (2020) let out that latitude, sunlight and vitamin D are possibly linked with increased COVID risks and its mortality. Tan *et al.* (2020) in Singapore supplemented vitamin D with magnesium and vitamin B_{12} on a small population suffering from the disease and reported the protective effect of this supplementation against COVID-19. Low vitamin D in European countries (except Nordic countries where people consume sufficient cod liver oil) especially during winter months is thought to be a reason behind the rapid spread of the disease during that period, though the finding needs further elucidation (Biesalski, 2020).

Vitamin D & COVID-19 and the Possible Mechanism Behind

Vitamin D which previously was thought to be only a vitamin but later it has been established as an important endocrine system. Primarily it is produced from 7-dehydrocholesterol in skin by the UV- radiation of sunlight. After going through some isomerisation cholecalciferol or vitamin D_3 is yielded. It is bound to carrier protein (vitamin D binding protein-VDB) and removed from skin. Both endogenous and exogenous vitamin D is metabolised mostly in liver and converted to 25-hydroxy cholecalciferol or 25(OH) vitamin D, major form of circulating vitamin D. Again it is converted to 1, 25 dihydroxy cholecalciferol mainly in kidney, the most active form of vitamin D which involves in various biological functions. It can also be produced in various other cells with 1-α hydroxylase enzyme activity; like in cells of immune system. Vitamin D Response which belongs to nuclear hormone receptor family is widely distributed in the body and upon binding with 1-25 dihydroxy vitamin D hetero-dimerization occurs with other such nuclear receptors, like member of Retinoid X receptor family. Such Complexes then bind to special DNA sequence, which is called Vitamin D Response Elements (VDRE) and regulate genetic expression thus exhibit classical or non-classical functions of this vitamin (Bikle, 2014). These might play significant protective role of vitamin D against COVID-19.

Immunomodulation and Vitamin D

Vitamin D modulates innate and adaptive immune system and also provides physical barrier to microbial infections. It plays following roles in this context-

• It maintains integrity of epithelial cells through regulating tight or gap junctions and induces cellular molecules like E-cadherin for binding cells at adherens junctions (Schwalfenberg, 2011).

- This vitamin mediates innate immunity either directly through the production of antimicrobial peptides or by inhibiting cytokine storm production by innate immune system.

- Vitamin D stimulates expression of antimicrobial peptides like cathelicdin, defensin, LL-37. Studies have already shown that cathelicdin is effective even against corona virus and can prevent lung injury due to hypoxia in COVID patients. These peptides can also arrest survival and replication of viruses. (Liu *et al.*, 2006; Jiang *et al.*, 2020)

- Body generates pro-inflammatory and anti-inflammatory cytokines through innate immunity in response to infection which is also seen in COVID-19. Vitamin D suppresses the expression of pro-inflammatory cytokines like TNF-α or interferon γ whereas up-regulates expression of anti-inflammatory cytokines (Grant *et al.*, 2020).

- Deficiency of vitamin D fails to mature macrophages or to present its specific surface antigens in response to microbial infection and also fails to produce H_2O_2, a potent anti-microbial agent via lysosomal enzyme acid phosphatase activity (Di Rosa *et al.*, 2011).

- It also regulates adaptive immunity via promoting the responses of T-helper cell type 2 (Th2) whereas suppresses the response of T-helper cell type 1(Th1) cells. Calcitriol also influence anti-inflammatory cytokine production by Th2 cells which has again an indirect effect to suppress Th1 immune response (Cantorna *et al.*, 2015).

- Vitamin D in many ways influences to up raise the anti-inflammatory cytokine production e.g. (interleukin or IL) IL3, IL4, IL5 or IL10 whereas level of pro-inflammatory cytokines are diminished like TNF-α, interferon γ, nuclear factor-kB (NF-kB) or IL-2, IL-6, IL-12 and IL-17, hs-CRP (high sensitivity C-reactive protein). These simultaneously subsides cytokine storm, a significant bio marker of COVID-19 (Prietl *et al.*, 2013; Aygun, 2020).

- Vitamin D helps to promote proliferation of T-reg (T regulatory) cells, thus reduces inflammation.

- It has proved to improve influenza by escalating serological response towards the vaccine and also influencing the function of CD8+. In COVID-19 altered function of T lymphocytes are found and lymphopenia is also common. It is thought vitamin D can improve disease severity through its role on CD8+ T cells (Teymoori-Rad and Marashi, 2020)

- Vitamin D supplementation has successfully enhanced CD4+ T helper cells in HIV infection but its influence in COVID-19 is still unknown (Alvarez *et al.*, 2019).

- It also limits leukocyte infiltration to the sites of inflammation.
- This vitamin interacts with other innate immune cells like neutrophils, lymphocytes, monocytes, macrophages, mast cells or dendritic cells as well. And it alters their ratio and control functions through which also exhibit immune modulation effects (Teymoori-Rad and Marashi, 2020).

Renin –Angiotensin System (RAS) and Vitamin D

- Hypovitaminosis of vitamin D increases renin activity; raises circulating Angiotensin II (Ang-II), which stimulates aldosterone secretion and simultaneous systemic vasoconstriction occurs, leading to hypertension – the most affected co morbidity in COVID-19 (Forman *et al.*, 2010)
- Angiotensin Converting Enzyme 2 (ACE2) of this system down regulates RAS activity by degradation of both Ang-I and Ang-II into Ang1-9 and Ang1-7 respectively and also inhibits ACE/Ang-II/ATR1 axis and related pro inflammatory cytokine synthesis; counterbalancing this activity via activation of ACE2/Ang1-9/AT2R and ACE2/Ang1-7/Mas axis (Aygun, 2020; Biesalski, 2020)
- Both vitamin D and ACE2 are the negative regulators of RAS which in turn down regulates pro-inflammatory cytokine production and maintains blood pressure as well. Supplementation of this vitamin is found beneficial in essential hypertension.
- Now in COVID-19 spike protein of SARS-COV-2 binds with ACE2 receptors and enters human cells. This up-regulates expression of metallo-peptidase ADAM17 which in turn down-regulates the expression and function of ACE2, thus leads to severe inflammation developing ARDS, lung, blood vessels or heart injuries. (Xu *et al.*, 2017; Biesalski, 2020; Kreutz *et al.*, 2020)
- Patients who are hypertensive, diabetic or patients with kidney disease receive RAS blocker drugs which over-express ACE2, make those people more susceptible for COVID19 and its severe complications. This can also be counter balanced by vitamin D as it down-regulates ACE2 expression and can prevent the virus entry (Arboleda and Urcuqui- Inchima, 2020).

DPP4/CD 26 Receptor and Vitamin D

- Recent findings have revealed that not only ACE2 receptors but the spikes protein of SARS-COV2 can also bind with dipeptidyl peptidase 4 (DPP4/CD26) receptors to enter the cells like previous MERS corona virus (Vankadari and Wilce, 2020)

- These co-receptors are also widely distributed in cell surface of vascular, epithelial cells in respiratory tract, lung, kidney, intestine and heart. (Meyerholz *et al.*, 2016)

- This invasion of virus into human cells via DPP4 triggers inflammation and produces cytokine storm leading to ARDS and other lung injuries.

- DPP4 is over-expressed in obese and people with diabetes and make those persons more susceptible to undergo severe COVID-19 outcomes.

- Interestingly vitamin D has a role to down regulate the expression of DPP4- another possible role to reduce the risk or severity of the disease (Komolmit *et al.*, 2017; McCartney and Byrne, 2020; Valencia *et al.*, 2020).

Cardio-protective Effect

- Now it is known to all severe outcomes of COVID-19 often includes endothelial damages, myocardial and other cardiac injuries. People with cardiovascular disease are more susceptible to get infected and to undergo the severity of COVID-19 (Zheng *et al.*, 2020). Dysregulated RAS, increased level of circulating DPP4 and improper expression of ACE2, all lead to inflammation which pre exist in cardio vascular diseases, aggravate disease condition (Valencia *et al.* 2020).

- Vitamin D has protective effect on endothelial cells and muscular cells of heart. Deficiency is a potent risk factor for developing cardio vascular disease, hypertension, and dyslipidemia.

- Deficiency also promotes vascular calcification, thickening of intima, ventricular hypertrophy, endothelial dysfunction, altered coagulation and increases pro inflammatory markers (Kunadian *et al.*, 2014; Verdoia and Luca, 2020).

- It has anti-oxidant, anti inflammatory and anti thrombogenic property. Vitamin D also inhibits atherosclerotic plaque formation. It hinders expression of PAI-1 i.e. Plasminogen Activator Inhibitor-1 and thrombospondin-1 whereas increases expression of thrombomodulin (Aihara *et al.*, 2004).

- Low Vitamin D activates RAS, concentrates Ang II, and increases Na^+ absorption, raises aldosterone level; Blood pressure enhances with insulin resistance, diabetes, cardio vascular disease (Biesalski, 2020).

- Nitric oxide (NO), which maintains normal vascular environment, also proved important for treating previous SARS infection, 2004. And it can even play pivotal role in SARS-COV2 infection, though its role is under clinical trial. This NO production is again modulated by vitamin D (Akerström *et al.*, 2020).

Pulmonary

- ACE2 knock out in experimental mice showed development of ARDS, a severe cause of COVID19 mortality (Imai *et al.*, 2005).

- Supplementation of vitamin D has proved to down regulating Renin/ACE/ AngII/AT1R cascade mechanism rather up regulates ACE2/Ang 1-7 pathway and prevents ARDS and lung injuries (Biesalski, 2020).

- Vitamin D also protects lungs against lipo polysaccharide induced lung damages (Xu *et al.* 2017).

- Anti inflammatory effect of this vitamin restrains 'cytokine storm' of COVID-19 (Biesalski, 2020).

- This vitamin found to be protective against interstitial pneumonia in experimental animal model, a clinical feature of COVID-19 severity.

- Deficiency of this vitamin is related with hypoxia, pulmonary oedema and sepsis (Dancer *et al.*, 2015; Verdoia and Luca, 2020).

Others

- Deficiency of vitamin D is a common feature of obesity. Obesity over activates RAS, decreases adiponectin secretion, increases inflammatory cytokines, incurs other co morbidities and such persons become 'at risk' for getting infected by SARS-COV2 and often suffer hard from this infection (Biesalski, 2020).

- Pre-diabetic and diabetic are the other co-morbidities which frequently get affected heavily by COVID-19 by the same ways involving dysregulated RAS, raised inflammatory cytokines, imbalanced expression of ACE2 and DPP4 (Suvarna and Mohan, 2020; Valencia *et al.*, 2020). This vitamin D improves insulin sensitivity and low serum concentration of this vitamin causes dysfunction of beta cells and insulin resistance which aggravate COVID-19 outcomes (Li and Zhou, 2015).

- SARS-COV 2 deletes host gene which is involved in expression of host's stress response and promotes inflammation. Vitamin D suppresses stress in Endoplasmic reticulum (ER) and also the oxidative stress in endothelial cells through its role on adhesion and migration of macrophages and or scavenging activities (De diego *et al.*, 2011; Sacco *et al.*, 2012).

- Vitamin D influences genetic expression of endogenous antioxidants like glutathione reductase, this spares vitamin C and let it act to preventing and treating microbial infection and related injuries (Wimalawansa, 2020).

VITAMIN D SUPPLEMENTATION IN COVID-19

Across the world countries like US, Brazil, Spain, Australia and many more are already investigating the therapeutic effect of supplementation of vitamin D on COVID-19 patients. Observational or interventional studies are going on to detect the impact of this vitamin on different stages of COVID-19. The possible mechanism, its effect on other respiratory infectious diseases and other co-morbidities of COVID-19 has made us to hypothesise that supplementation of vitamin D might be cost effective, safe and easily accessible therapeutic agent to treat COVID-19 or protect against this disease. But more studies are required to throw light on the possible risks, disadvantages or the dosage of vitamin D to be administered on patients with COVID-19 (Arboleda and Urcuqui-Inchima, 2020;Tey moori-Rad and Marashi, 2020).

Recommended Dietary Allowance (RDA) of Vitamin D and its Rich Sources

For the Indians the RDA for vitamin D is 400 I.U/day for adults. During this pandemic era, home confinement during lock down or coming winter days in India or pre existing vitamin D deficiency could make a person susceptible for the disease and its worst outcomes. Though this vitamin is readily available from endogenous source but it can also be achieved from exogenous rich sources, which include cod liver oil, mushroom, egg yolk, animal liver, sea fish and also milk and their products are fair sources of this vitamin (Srilakshmi, 2014).

CONCLUSION

From the above discussion it is clear that vitamin D deficiency is a pandemic, affecting billions of people across the world. It is also a potent immunomodulator, antimicrobial, anti-inflammatory and antioxidant agent; that has been successfully supplemented to combat several communicable and non communicable diseases as well. Though more studies and clinical trials are to be done regarding the therapeutic usage of vitamin D supplementation in different stages of COVID-19, but it is clear that low serum concentration of this vitamin is definitely a potent risk factor to aggravate the disease condition. So, people with vitamin D deficiency can have some vitamin D enriched foods to upraise its serum concentration and also to boost up our immune system.

REFERENCES

Aihara K, Azuma H, Akaike M, *et al.* (2004) Disruption of nuclear vitamin D receptor gene causes enhanced thrombogenicity in mice. *J Biol Chem* **279(34)**:35798-35802.

Akerström S, Mousavi-Jazi M, Klingström J, Leijon M, Lundkvist A, Mirazimi A (2005) Nitric oxide inhibits the replication cycle of severe acute respiratory syndrome coronavirus. *J Virol* **79(3):** 1966-1969.

Ali N (2020) Role of vitamin D in preventing of COVID-19 infection, progression and severity. *J Infect Public Health* S1876–0341 doi 10.1016/ j.jiph.2020.06.021

Alvarez N, Aguilar-Jimenez W, Rugeles MT (2019) The Potential Protective Role of Vitamin D Supplementation on HIV-1 Infection. *Front Immunol* **10:** 2291.

Aparna P, Muthathal S, Nongkynrih B, Gupta SK (2018) Vitamin D deficiency in India. *J Family Med Prim Care* **7:** 324-30.

Arboleda JF, Urcuqui-Inchima S (2020) Vitamin D Supplementation: A Potential Approach for Coronavirus/COVID-19 Therapeutics? *Front Immunol* **11:** 1523.

Aygun H (2020) Vitamin D can prevent COVID-19 infection-induced multiple organ damage. *Naunyn-Schmiedeberg's Arch Pharmacol* **393:** 1157–1160.

Biesalski HK (2020) Vitamin D deficiency and co-morbidities in COVID-19 patients – A fatal relationship? *Nfs Journal* **20:** 10-21.

Bikle DD (2014) Vitamin D metabolism, mechanism of action, and clinical applications. *Chem Biol* **21(3):** 319–329.

Burrell C, Howard C, Murphy F (2016) Fenner and White's Medical Virology (5th Edn). Academic, USA.

Cantorna MT, Snyder L, Lin YD, Yang L (2015) Vitamin D and 1,25(OH)2D regulation of T cells. Nutrients **7:** 3011–3021.

Centers for Disease Control and Prevention (11 Sept, 2020) Coronavirus Disease 2019 (COVID-19): People with certain medical conditions. Web. https:// www.cdc.gov/coronavirus/2019-ncov/need-extra-precautions/people-with-medical-conditions.html

Chen N, Zhou M, Dong X, *et al* (2020) Epidemiological and clinical characteristics of 99 cases of 2019 novel coronavirus pneumonia in Wuhan, China: a descriptive study. *Lancet* **395(10223):** 507-513.

Dancer RC, Parekh D, Lax S, *et al* (2015) Vitamin D deficiency contributes directly to the acute respiratory distress syndrome (ARDS) *Thorax* **70(7):** 617-624.

Daneshkhah A, Agrawal V, Eshein A, *et al.* (2020) The Possible Role of Vitamin D in Suppressing Cytokine Storm and Associated Mortality in COVID-19 Patients. medRxiv. doi 10.1101/2020.04.08.20058578.

DeDiego ML, Nieto Torres JL, Jiménez Guardeño JM, *et al (2011)* severe acute respiratory syndrome coronavirus envelope protein regulates cell stress response and apoptosis. *PLoS Pathog. 7(10):e1002315.*

Di Rosa M, Malaguarnera M, Nicoletti F, Malaguarnera L (2011) Vitamin D3: a helpful immuno-modulator. *Immunology* **134(2):** 123-139.

Forman JP, Williams JS, Fisher ND (2010) Plasma 25-hydroxyvitamin D and regulation of the renin-angiotensin system in humans. *Hypertension* **55(5):** 1283-1288.

Graedel L, Merker M, Felder S, Kutz A, Haubitz S, Faessler L, Kaeslin M, Huber A, Mueller B, Schuetz P (2016) Vitamin D deficiency strongly predicts adverse medical outcome across different medical inpatient populations: results from a prospective study. *Medicine* **95(19):** e3533.

Grant WB, Lahore H, McDonnell SL, *et al* (2020) Evidence that Vitamin D Supplementation Could Reduce Risk of Influenza and COVID-19 Infections and Deaths. *Nutrients* **12(4):** 988.

Harapan H, Itoh N, Yufika A, *et al* (2020) Coronavirus disease 2019 (COVID-19): A literature review. *J Infect Public Health* **13(5):** 667-673.

Hastie CE, Mackay DF, Ho F, *et al* (2020) Vitamin D concentrations and COVID-19 infection in UK Biobank . *Diabetes Metab Syndr* **14(4):** 561-565

Holick MF, Binkley NC, Bischoff-Ferrari HA, Gordon CM, Hanley DA, Heaney RP, Murad MH, Weaver CM (2011) Evaluation, treatment, and prevention of vitamin D deficiency: an Endocrine Society clinical practice guideline. *J Clin Endocrinol Metab* **96(7):** 1911-30.

Huang C, Wang Y, Li X *et al.* (2020) Clinical features of patients infected with 2019 novel coronavirus in Wuhan, China. *Lancet* **395(10223):** 497-506.

Hui DS, I Azhar E, Madani TA, *et al.* (2020) The continuing 2019-nCoV epidemic threat of novel coronaviruses to global health - The latest 2019 novel coronavirus outbreak in Wuhan, China. *Int J Infect Dis* **91:** 264-266.

Imai Y, Kuba K, Rao S, *et al* (2005) Angiotensin-converting enzyme 2 protects from severe acute lung failure. *Nature* **436(7047):** 112-116.

Jiang JS, Chou HC, Chen CM (2020) Cathelicidin attenuates hyperoxia-induced lung injury by inhibiting oxidative stress in newborn rats. *Free Radic Biol Med* **150:** 23-29.

Komolmit P, Charoensuk K, Thanapirom K *et al* (2017) Correction of vitamin D deficiency facilitated suppression of IP-10 and DPP IV levels in patients with chronic hepatitis C: A randomised double-blinded, placebo-control trial. *PLoS One* **12(4):** e0174608.

Kreutz R, Algharably EAE, Azizi M, *et al* (2020) Hypertension, the renin-angiotensin system, and the risk of lower respiratory tract infections and lung injury: implications for COVID-19. *Cardiovasc Res* **116(10):** 1688-1699.

Kunadian V, Ford GA, Bawamia B, Qiu W, Manson JE (2014) Vitamin D deficiency and coronary artery disease: a review of the evidence. *Am Heart J* **167(3):** 283-291.

Li F (2015) Receptor recognition mechanisms of coronaviruses: a decade of structural studies. *J Virol.* **89(4):** 1954-1964.

Li Y, Li Q, Zhang N, Liu Z (2020) Sunlight and vitamin D in the prevention of coronavirus disease (COVID-19) infection and mortality in the United States. Research Square doi: 10.21203/rs.3.rs-32499/v1.

Li YX, Zhou L (2015) Vitamin D deficiency, obesity and diabetes. *Cell Mol Biol* **61:**35–38.

Liu PT, Stenger S, Li H, *et al.* (2006) Toll-like receptor triggering of a vitamin D-mediated human antimicrobial response. *Science* **311(5768):** 1770-1773.

Lu R, Zhao X, Li J, Niu P, *et al.* (2020) Genomic characterisation and epidemiology of 2019 novel coronavirus: implications for virus origins and receptor binding. *Lancet* **395(10224):** 565-574.

Martineau AR, Forouhi NG (2020) Vitamin D for COVID-19: a case to answer? *Lancet Diabetes Endocrinol* **8(9):** 735-736.

McCartney DM, Byrne DG (2020) Optimisation of Vitamin D Status for Enhanced Immuno-protection Against Covid-19. *Ir Med J* **113(4):** 58.

Meyerholz DK, Lambertz AM, McCray PB (2016) Dipeptidyl Peptidase 4 Distribution in the Human Respiratory Tract: Implications for the Middle East Respiratory Syndrome. *Am J Pathol* **186(1):** 78-86.

Palacios C, Gonzalez L (2014) Is vitamin D deficiency a major global public health problem? *J Steroid Biochem Mol Biol* **144 Pt A:** 138-45.

Prietl B, Treiber G, Pieber TR, Amrein K (2013) Vitamin D and Immune Function. *Nutrients* **5:** 2502-2521.

Quraishi SA, De Pascale G, Needleman JS, *et al* (2015) Effect of Cholecalciferol Supplementation on Vitamin D Status and Cathelicidin Levels in Sepsis: A Randomized, Placebo-Controlled Trial. *Crit Care Med* **43(9):** 1928-1937.

Richman DD, Whitley RJ, Hayden FG (2016) Clinical Virology (4th Edn). ASM, Washington.

Sacco RE, Nonnecke BJ, Palmer MV, Waters WR, Lippolis JD, Reinhardt TA (2012) Differential expression of cytokines in response to respiratory syncytial virus infection of calves with high or low circulating 25-hydroxyvitamin D3. *PLoS One* **7(3):** e33074.

Schwalfenberg GK (2011) A review of the critical role of vitamin D in the functioning of the immune system and the clinical implications of vitamin D deficiency. *Mol Nutr Food Res* **55(1):** 96-108.

Singhal T (2020) A review of coronavirus Disease-2019 (COVID-19). *Indian J Pediatr* **87:** 281–286.

Srilakshmi B (2014) Nutrition Science (4th Edn). New Age International (P) limited, New Delhi.

Suvarna VR, Mohan V (2020) Vitamin D and its role in coronavirus disease 2019 (COVID-19). *J Diabetol* **11(2):** 71-80.

Tan CW, Ho LP, Kalimuddin S *et al* (2020) A cohort study to evaluate the effect of combination Vitamin D, Magnesium and Vitamin B12 (DMB) on progression to severe outcome in older COVID-19 patients. medRxiv doi:10.1101/ 2020.06.01.20112334 (Preprint)

Teymoori-Rad M, Marashi SM (2020) Vitamin D and Covid-19: From potential therapeutic effects to unanswered questions. *Rev Med Virol* e2159. https:// doi.org/10.1002/rmv.2159

Trovas G, Tournis S (2020) Vitamin D and covid-19. *Hormones (Athens)* **14:** 1– 2

Unhale S, Bilal Q, Sanap S, Thakhre S, Wadatkar S, Bairagi R, Sagrule S, Biyani KR (2020) A Review on Corona Virus (COVID-19). *Int J Pharm Life Sci* **6:** 109 - 115.

Valencia I, Peiró C, Lorenzo Ó, Sánchez-Ferrer CF, Eckel J, Romacho T(2020) DPP4 and ACE2 in Diabetes and COVID-19: Therapeutic Targets for Cardiovascular Complications? *Front Pharmacol* **11:** 1161.

Vankadari N, Wilce JA (2020) Emerging Wuhan (COVID-19) coronavirus: glycan shield and structure prediction of spike glycoprotein and its interaction with human CD26. *Emerg Microbes Infect.* **9(1):** 601-604.

Verdoia M, De Luca G (2020) Potential role of hypovitaminosis D and Vitamin D supplementation during COVID-19 pandemic. *QJM* **hcaa 234**. doi:10.1093/ qjmed/hcaa234

Wang C, Horby PW, Hayden FG, Gao GF (2020) A novel corona virus outbreak of global health concern. *Lancet* **395(10223):** 470-473.

Wimalawansa SJ (2020) Global epidemic of coronavirus—COVID-19: What we can do to minimize risks. Eur. J. Biomed. Pharm. Sci 7: 432–438.

World Health Organization (11March, 2020) WHO Director-General's opening remarks at the media briefing on COVID-19.Web. https://www.who.int/dg/speeches/detail/who-director-general-s-opening-remarks-at-the-media-briefing-on-covid-19—11-march-2020

World Health Organization (23 August, 2020) Corona Virus Disease (COVID-19). Web. https://covid19.who.int/?gclid=Cj0KCQjwp4j6BRCRARIsAGq4yMG0fMwYZGx70qPloNArSAZ9eEhzZc2b5lFJRSXeCNrz5r-g-xajhp0aAvKSEALw_wcB

World Health Organization (23 August, 2020) Web. https://covid19.who.int/region/searo/country/in

Xu J, Yang J, Chen J, Luo Q, Zhang Q, Zhang H (2017) Vitamin D alleviates lipopolysaccharide-induced acute lung injury via regulation of the renin-angiotensin system. *Mol Med Rep* **16:**7432–8.

Zheng Y, Ma Y, Zhang J, *et al* (2020) COVID-19 and the cardiovascular system. *Nat Rev Cardiol* **17:** 259–260.